W9-AXQ-042

R.A.D.L.
241 East Federal Highway
P.O. Box 888
Roscommon, MI 48653

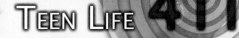

IT'S CANCER.

NOW WHAT?

LUKE GRAHAM
AND
HENRIETTA M. LILY

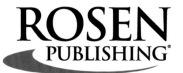

ROSEN
PUBLISHING®

New York

Published in 2012 by The Rosen Publishing Group, Inc.
29 East 21st Street, New York, NY 10010

Copyright © 2012 by The Rosen Publishing Group, Inc.

First Edition

All rights reserved. No part of this book may be reproduced in any form without permission in writing from the publisher, except by a reviewer.

Library of Congress Cataloging-in-Publication Data

Graham, Luke.
It's cancer: now what? / Luke Graham, Henrietta M. Lily.
    p. cm.—(Teen life 411)
Includes bibliographical references and index.
ISBN 978-1-4488-4652-8 (library binding)
1. Cancer—Popular works. I. Lily, Henrietta M. II. Title.
RC263.G697 2012
616.99'4—dc22

2010042036

Manufactured in the United States of America

CPSIA Compliance Information: Batch #S11YA: For further information, contact Rosen Publishing, New York, New York, at 1-800-237-9932.

CONTENTS

INTRODUCTION...4

CHAPTER 1 WHAT CANCER IS AND HOW IT WORKS...7

CHAPTER 2 HOW THE HUMAN BODY FIGHTS DISEASE: THE IMMUNE SYSTEM IN ACTION...16

CHAPTER 3 CANCER TRIGGERS AND RISK FACTORS...23

CHAPTER 4 IMPROVING THE ODDS: REDUCING THE LIKELIHOOD OF CANCER...34

CHAPTER 5 SCREENING AND TESTING FOR CANCER...54

CHAPTER 6 CONFRONTING THE WORST: COPING WITH A DIAGNOSIS OF CANCER...63

CHAPTER 7 TYPES OF CANCER TREATMENT...86

CHAPTER 8 WHEN TREATMENT FAILS...112

CHAPTER 9 LIFE AFTER CANCER TREATMENT...119

ABOUT DR. JAN...129
GLOSSARY...130
FOR MORE INFORMATION...134
FOR FURTHER READING...138
INDEX...140

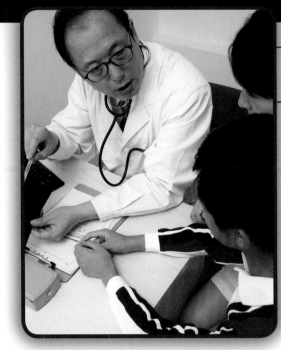

In past generations, people worried about being stricken by diseases like tuberculosis, smallpox, and cholera. These were illnesses that were often deadly. One of the goals of the medical profession is to solve the riddle of such diseases and find new and more effective ways of preventing, diagnosing, treating, and even eradicating them. Today, people are not as afraid of tuberculosis, smallpox, or cholera because the medical profession has found ways to prevent and effectively treat these diseases.

Sometimes, the medical profession has to keep looking for answers on certain kinds of illness. Even after years of research and experimentation, cures and treatments for certain diseases remain elusive or not as effective as hoped. Cancer is one of those illnesses. Cancer treatment and research can be traced back to ancient Egypt, about 1600 BCE. Cancer was—and is—a mystifying disease.

A doctor explains a boy's diagnosis to him and his mother.

It was not until the early twentieth century that some cancer treatments finally began to prove effective. These newer treatments were considered successful because some patients were cured. However, cancer stubbornly persists. It remains a disease that most people dread, even though the rate of successful treatment outcomes has risen even as mortality rates have fallen.

Researchers are still hard at work looking for better ways to prevent, diagnose, and treat cancer. The science that they practice is called oncology, and they are referred to as oncologists. New methods or technologies for researching cancer are also being developed. With ever-greater advances in science and technology, answers to questions about cancer are becoming increasingly clear and detailed.

Even though cancer is slowly being demystified and treated more effectively, most people still become afraid when they hear the word "cancer." Fear of the disease has been so great that it was not until the late twentieth century that people were willing to talk about cancer in public. Some people still consider the subject taboo. When people are afraid to talk about a certain subject, it keeps the facts from being known. Superstition and misinformation take the place of actual and useful knowledge. In many cases, the lack of knowledge about cancer has caused unnecessary grief and fear. Often what people imagine about cancer is far worse than the actual prognosis or outcome.

One of the most important things to remember about cancer is that it is OK to talk about it. We no longer have to be afraid of the word, and we certainly should not be afraid of anyone who has—or had—cancer. It's important to seek answers to questions about cancer because as more is learned, more knowledge will be gained. The more knowledge one is armed with, the less there is to fear.

This book will cover topics relating to cancer, including causes, prevention, diagnosis, and treatment. If you know someone with cancer or have it yourself, the best thing to do is to learn more about it. The more you know, the less helpless you or a loved one will feel during the difficult time of being diagnosed and treated. Many cancer patients have said that once they learned more about the disease, they felt more in control of what was happening to them.

Even if you do not know anyone with cancer, it is still important that you learn about it. Someone you know, or you yourself, may be at risk for developing certain cancers or may be diagnosed with cancer someday. There are things that anyone can do—starting right now—to greatly lower his or her risk of developing certain kinds of cancers. Knowing the facts about the causes of certain cancers and the risks associated with them is important. It can help you avoid engaging in activities that increase your chances of developing certain kinds of cancer. You can also help your loved ones avoid these cancer-causing activities.

One of the reasons why cancer remains challenging to researchers is that it is not a single disease. The word "cancer" is used to describe more than one hundred different diseases. Some cancers are very serious, while others are almost never life threatening. Many cancers fall somewhere in between. Each kind of cancer has its own name. Cancers behave differently in different individuals. Some develop very quickly, whereas others develop very slowly. Different cancers are treated in different ways, and the results from these treatments vary from person to person. However, all of the various cancers have one thing in common: the process of how they begin to grow and develop in the body.

THE MECHANICS OF CANCER

Cancer begins at the cellular level. That means it starts to develop in the body's cells. There are trillions of tiny cells that make up the human body. It is important to know, however, that just because the human body is made up of so many cells, it is not inevitable that some of them will become cancerous.

There are many different types of cells, each with a specialized job to perform in the body. The human body experiences daily wear and tear that damages the cells. New cells are

WHAT CANCER IS AND HOW IT WORKS

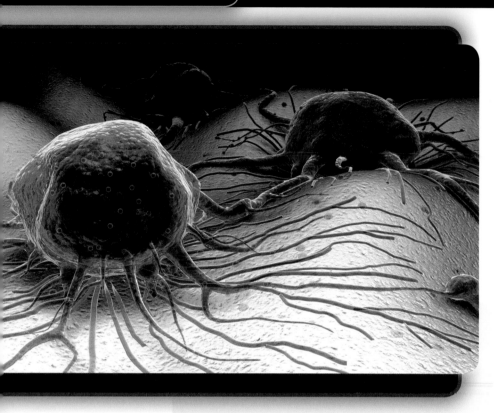

A scanning electron microscopic image reveals cancer cells developing on the surface of healthy tissue.

needed to replace old, damaged cells. In order to make
new cells, each cell divides in two. Ordinarily, cells divide
and produce more cells only when the body needs them.
Cells get their directions to divide from genes. Genes
control several different functions of the cells. This process of new cell creation and the replacement of old cells
is how the human body stays healthy and strong.

Cancer starts when a few cells of the body go haywire by dividing out of control. A cancer cell divides even
when new cells are not needed. A cell that goes haywire

is an abnormal cell. Abnormal cells grow more quickly than normal cells. When the abnormal cells keep dividing, a mass of tissue forms. Tissue is a collection of cells that perform a specific function. The tissue that is formed from abnormal cells, however, does not have a function. The tissue made by abnormal, cancerous cells is abnormal, too.

The tissue that is formed from abnormal cells is called a tumor. Other names for a tumor are growth, lump, or neoplasm. The good news is that not all tumors are cancerous. If you find a lump, definitely talk to a parent and doctor about it, but also know that most lumps are not cancerous.

The term "tumor" was once used to describe any swelling. Now it's used to describe any abnormal mass of tissue. Tumors can develop in almost any part of the body. They are classified as either benign or malignant.

BENIGN TUMORS

Benign literally means "to be of a gentle nature," to be harmless. Benign tumors grow slowly and stay in one place. The cells of this kind of tumor do not invade nearby tissues or organs. They keep dividing and making abnormal tissue, but they do not spread; they keep to themselves. Many of us live with benign tumors or growths without even knowing it. Examples of common benign tumors are moles and warts on the skin.

Even though benign tumors are not cancerous, they still have the potential to interfere with the normal functioning of the body. Benign tumors may grow large

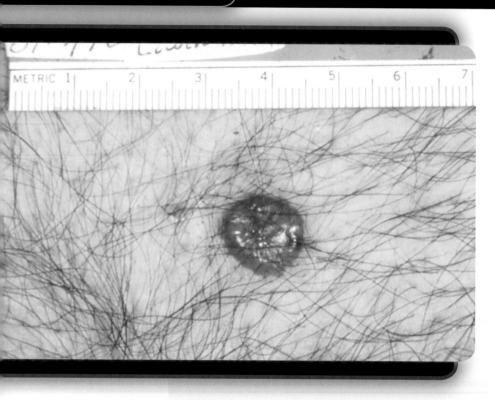

This tumor is a basal cell carcinoma, a form of skin cancer. They are often small, reddish-brown or translucent and pearly, with a depression at the center.

enough to crowd other cells and tissues. If they grow too large, they can be surgically removed. After removal, benign tumors rarely grow back. Some are completely harmless and thus need no treatment at all. Here are some other types of benign tumors:

- **Abscesses.** These are collections of pus that are usually caused by a bacterial infection. Surface abscesses are called boils. Abscesses frequently occur in moist areas of the body, such as the groin or armpits.

- **Cysts.** These are abnormal swellings or sacs that usually contain fluid. Cysts can occur in almost any body tissue. They are most frequently found in the skin, female breasts, and ovaries.
- **Fibroids.** These are solid growths. They can appear in or around the uterus. Fibroids are made mostly of muscle tissue.
- **Polyps.** These are growths that develop in the lining of certain organs. Polyps may occur anywhere in the body but are most common in the nose, colon, and uterus. They are usually benign, but sometimes a polyp is found to be precancerous, which means that it is in the early stages of becoming cancer.

MALIGNANT TUMORS

Malignant means "to cause harm." Malignant tumors usually grow rapidly. Malignant cells can invade and destroy nearby tissues and organs. They can also spread to other parts of the body by a process called metastasis. During metastasis, tumor cells break away and form secondary tumors elsewhere in the body. The cells usually travel to other parts of the body by breaking into a blood vessel or a lymphatic vessel. These vessels operate like highways in the body, allowing the tumors to travel and develop elsewhere.

The shape of a malignant tumor often resembles that of a crab, which is how cancer gets its name. The word "cancer" is Latin for "crab." There are more than a hundred types of cancers that can afflict the human body. Most of them belong to one of four major tissue types:

- **Carcinomas.** These develop in the epithelial tissue. Epithelial tissue is the covering of external and internal body parts. Skin is epithelial tissue. So is the tissue that lines or covers internal organs. Carcinomas also develop in the body's glandular cells. Carcinomas are the most common kinds of cancer. They are most often found in the skin, colon, stomach, lungs, and prostate gland.
- **Leukemias.** These are cancers of the blood cells. They are found in the bloodstream and in blood-forming tissues (bone marrow and the spleen).
- **Lymphomas.** These are found in the organs of the lymphatic and immune system. These organs, which produce and store infection-fighting cells, include the lymph nodes, spleen, and thymus. Infection-fighting cells are in almost all tissues of the body, which makes other organs (like the tonsils or stomach) more vulnerable to lymphomas.
- **Sarcomas.** These develop in the connective or supportive tissues of the body. This tissue includes the cartilage, joints, bones, tendons, muscles, blood vessels, and body fat.

How Cancers Are Named

The names of some cancers are very long, such as "adenocarcinoma." If you break the name into parts,

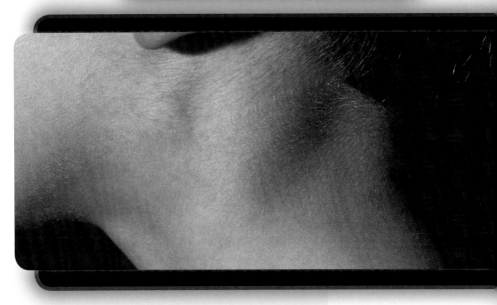

This boy has a swollen lymph node on the side of his neck. Swollen lymph nodes usually indicate infection, but in some cases they can be a symptom of cancer. All swollen nodes and glands should be seen by a doctor.

it may be easier to understand. *Adeno* means "gland." Carcinoma is one of the four main types of cancers. Adenocarcinoma is a cancer of a gland. Other examples are osteosarcoma (bone cancer) and liposarcoma (cancer of fat cells). Here are some other prefixes that form part of a cancer's name and indicate its location:

- Chrondo-: cartilage
- Erythro-: red blood cells
- Hemangio-: blood vessels
- Hepato-: liver
- Lipo-: fat

CANCER FACTS

- The five-year survival rate (five years after diagnosis) for all cancers is now nearly 70 percent. From 1975 to 1977, the five-year survival rate was only 50 percent. This dramatic improvement is attributed to earlier diagnosis and improvements in treatment.
- Successfully treated patients often lead long, productive lives after being treated for cancer. Many are considered to be cured permanently.
- Cancer is not contagious; it cannot be caught from someone else.
- Cancer is not caused by an injury, such as a bruise or broken bone.
- Cancer is not a punishment upon the person who gets it for some sin or lifestyle choice; neither is cancer treatment. Cancer is a disease with complex causes and unpredictable progressions, but it is not a judgment upon the patient.
- If someone in a family has cancer, it does not necessarily mean that other people in the family will also develop it.
- There are many different kinds of cancer—affecting various parts of the body—and several stages of cancer, each with its own average survival rates. For this reason, many doctors are starting to use the term "cancers," rather than the singular word "cancer."
- Pain is not a typical symptom of early forms of most cancers. Therefore, the presence or absence of pain cannot be taken as a reliable early warning sign of disease.
- There are some cancers that can be prevented by things that we do or don't do, such as avoiding smoking, chewing tobacco, sun exposure, and excessive alcohol consumption, and maintaining a healthy weight and following a balanced, low-fat diet rich in fruits and vegetables and featuring whole grains and lean protein.

- Lympho-: lymphocyte (white blood cells)
- Melano-: pigment cells (skin cells)
- Myelo-: bone cells
- Myo-: muscle
- Osteo-: bone

Cancers can also be named for the organ they affect, such as lung cancer, stomach cancer, liver cancer, and breast cancer.

WHEN SWELLING IS NOT A LUMP

From time to time, a person may notice one or more swollen lumps along his or her armpits, neck, or groin. These lumps are most likely swollen lymph nodes. Lymph nodes, also known as lymph glands, are small, oval structures. They are part of the lymphatic and immune systems. The immune system responds to infections and foreign substances by trapping bacteria and other foreign and invasive disease-causing particles in the lymph nodes, where they are attacked and destroyed by infection-fighting cells. The lymph nodes swell when they are fighting infection and can feel like lumps just under the skin.

Swollen lymph glands can cause pain and tenderness during colds, flu, ear infections, and sore throats. They can also swell when a person's body is fighting diseases such as mononucleosis ("mono"), some cancers, and HIV infection (HIV is the virus that causes AIDS). To be absolutely safe, any swellings on the body should be shown to a parent, nurse, or doctor.

CHAPTER 2

The human body is constantly exposed to germs, viruses, and parasites. Bacteria and viruses are in the air, on the things that we eat and drink, on everything that we touch, and even on our skin. Germs are tiny infection-causing organisms that want to invade the body. They want to enter the body because it provides a good place for them to grow. The body would be a great place for germs to grow if it weren't for the immune system. Without the immune system, germs would grow uncontrolled, using the body as a host.

DETECTING FOREIGN INVADERS

The cells of the immune system scan the entire body to identify the presence of foreign substances. Cells and substances that are natural to the body have molecules (tiny parts) the immune system cells recognize. The molecules basically tell the immune system that these substances are part of the body's own cells. The molecules send a "self" signal. An invading infectious substance has foreign molecules

White blood cells *(blue in this image)* surround a measles virus. These cells are the infection fighters of the immune system. They stick to the surface of viruses and other foreign invaders and signal to other immune cells to attack.

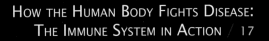

that the immune system doesn't recognize. These molecules send a "nonself" signal. Immune cells attack anything that sends a nonself signal. The immune system's army of infection-fighting white blood cells moves in to eliminate or kill the intruder.

The immune army is made of lymphocytes and many other kinds of white blood cells. These cells are located throughout the body and work together to fight foreign infectious substances. Lymphocytes make substances known as antibodies. Antibodies attack and destroy foreign substances that invade the body.

COMPROMISING THE IMMUNE SYSTEM

A person's immune system can be strong or weak. A number of factors can affect its strength. The genes that a person inherits can influence the immune system. Illnesses that a person has already been exposed to can weaken or strengthen the immune system. For example, an HIV infection can weaken the immune system and invite other illnesses. Yet someone who has been infected by the chicken pox virus receives immunity from it and usually cannot be infected again. If a person's immune system is weak, he or she can develop very serious illnesses much more easily than a person with a strong and healthy immune system will. Things that hurt or compromise the strength of the immune system should be avoided. Likewise, there are things that can be done to strengthen the immune system and increase its ability to fight off invasive attacks by bacteria and viruses.

Conditions or behaviors that can damage the body's immune system, thereby lowering its resistance to disease, include:

- Infectious agents, such as viruses, bacteria, or parasites
- Excessive alcohol consumption
- The taking of certain drugs and medications
- Lack of sleep
- Stress
- Depression
- Loneliness or isolation
- Overeating
- Malnutrition
- Exposure to allergens, such as those found in pollen, dust, or certain foods
- Vitamin deficiencies
- Exposure to air and water pollution
- Undergoing certain cancer treatments

STRENGTHENING THE IMMUNE SYSTEM

Conditions or behaviors that are believed to strengthen the body's immune system, thereby increasing its resistance to disease, include:

Power Up!

In a laboratory setting, cells of the immune system can actually kill cancerous tumor cells. Also, studies indicate that cancer patients have a better outcome when their immune system is at its strongest. The outcome is most favorable when the number of infection-fighting cells is at its highest. A strong immune system response may also be the reason why cancer can suddenly disappear from the body of a patient.

In addition to its likely role in fighting or preventing cancer, a strong immune system is essential for general good health. The human body is healthiest when its immune system is strong. The body is able to withstand exposure to many germs, viruses, and bacteria without being seriously damaged in the process.

- Healthy diet
- Avoiding drug and tobacco use and excessive alcohol consumption
- Getting enough sleep
- Proper hygiene
- Positive attitude
- Laughter
- Regular physical exercise
- Vitamins
- Meditation
- Relaxation and deep breathing techniques

Research suggests that in addition to responding to invading infectious substances, the immune system can also attack emerging and growing cancer cells. Immunologists—doctors who specialize in the study and treatment of the immune system—believe that the immune system does so on a regular basis. They believe that cancer cells develop on a regular basis but that the immune system suppresses or eliminates most of them before they can form a tumor and spread. Immunologists think that cancer has an opportunity to take hold and tumors develop only when the immune system is weak. It is still not understood how the immune system works to suppress cancer and why it

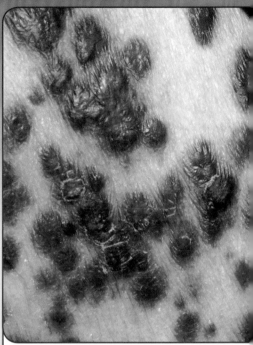

The skin of an AIDS patient is covered with Kaposi's sarcoma tumors. This is a kind of cancer caused by a herpes virus, and it can afflict those with weakened immune systems.

sometimes fails to do so. The link between cancer and the immune system is also suggested by the fact that people with AIDS, which is characterized primarily by a weakened immune system, are more likely to develop certain cancers.

As with invading bacteria and viruses, the immune system will attack cancer cells when they are identified as nonself substances. This does not always happen, however, because cancer cells originate from cells that are part of the body, not foreign invaders. The immune system sees the cancer cells as self, even though these cells are harmful. However, there are proteins within cancer cells that can send a nonself signal. The immune system will respond against the cancer when the nonself signals are active. Scientists are hard at work trying to locate the proteins that send nonself signals from within cancer cells. This may someday lead to more efficient and effective—and less painful and destructive—treatments against cancer.

CHAPTER 3

Different types of cancer take different amounts of time to develop. It can take anywhere from five to forty years for a tumor to go through the entire process of becoming large enough to produce symptoms. This long and slow development period is one of the reasons why it has been difficult to find one clear answer regarding what causes cancer. However, after many years of research, two main factors that allow cells to become cancerous have been identified:

- The cells that grow abnormally have a predisposition, or tendency, to grow abnormally. Something inside of the cells allows or instructs them to grow out of control.
- Damage or other external influences can cause healthy cells to become cancerous. The most important of these external influences are carcinogens, which are toxic, cancer-causing agents.

EXTERNAL INFLUENCES

Researchers and doctors agree that people can develop cancer through repeated, long-term contact with one or more carcinogens. It is estimated that up to 80 percent of all cancers are connected to carcinogens from the following:

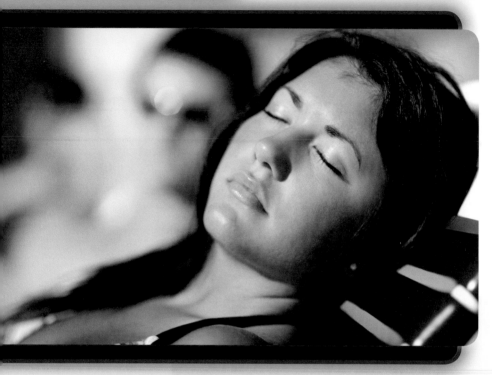

Limiting exposure to sun and wearing sunscreen that includes UVA and UVB protection and a high sun protection factor (SPF) can drastically reduce one's chances of developing skin cancer.

- Tobacco products (cigarettes, cigars, and chew)
- Overexposure to radiation (X-ray machines, uranium, radon, nuclear emissions, cancer treatments)
- Overexposure to sunlight (UV rays and visible light)
- Certain foods, drinks, and medications (excessive alcohol consumption, the consuming of charred foods, and the taking of some cholesterol-lowering drugs)
- The environment and the workplace (chemicals and solvents)

GENETIC PREDISPOSITION TO CANCER

A number of cancers develop through a combination of predisposition and exposure to cancer-causing agents. An example of this would be a comparison between two lifelong smokers. One of the one-pack-a-day smokers developed lung cancer, while the other smoker did not, even though he smoked the same amount over the same period of time. The smoker who developed lung cancer may have had cells that already had a predisposition or tendency to grow abnormally. Under this theory, the carcinogens in tobacco serve as a triggering agent for the cells to become cancerous. This does not mean that the other smoker was not being exposed to carcinogens. It just means that his cells had less of a preexisting tendency to become cancerous.

The tendency or predisposition that a cell has to turn cancerous is classified as either high or low. There is either a high tendency or a low tendency for the cells to become cancerous. Cells with a high tendency turn cancerous more easily than cells with a low tendency. The cells with a high tendency need very little exposure to carcinogens in order to become cancerous, whereas cells with a low tendency can handle more exposure to carcinogens. It is also possible that a person will develop cancer regardless of the degree of his or her exposure to carcinogens.

ASK DR. JAN, PSYCHOLOGIST

First Name: Anonymous

Question:
My grandmother died of breast cancer and an aunt is a breast cancer survivor. So I think I probably have a genetic predisposition to breast cancer. This is something I think and worry about every day. It's always in the back of my mind. How can I be proactive about my health instead of feeling like I'm waiting around for the inevitable bad news. Or how can I at least learn how to deal with this constant anxiety?

Answer:
While it is true that having one or more, particularly first-degree (mother, sister, daughter) relatives diagnosed with breast cancer increases your risk, it still doesn't mean that you will develop breast cancer. Consider the difference of probable stress of these two statements: "Because my grandmother and aunt had breast cancer, I will probably have it, too," and "Just because my grandmother and aunt had breast cancer doesn't mean that I definitely will." The first statement, which is not really factual, will generate a lot more anxiety than the second statement, which is based in fact. The point here is that there are things that are potentially within your control, like your thinking, which can help reduce your stress level about this issue. The truth is that even if you are unfortunate enough to ever get breast cancer, it would still be to your advantage to live life now and in the future to its fullest.

While there are no guaranteed ways to prevent breast cancer, you can reduce some known risk factors by avoiding excessive weight gain or obesity, exercising regularly, and minimizing the use of alcohol. Studies also suggest that women who breast-feed for a long period of time reduce their risk of breast cancer.

Most experts agree that it is also important to have regular medical checkups that include a clinical breast examination and mammograms, when recommended by your doctor.

Ask a Question

Do you have a question that you would like answered? E-mail your question to Dr. Jan at drjan@rosenpub.com. If your question is selected, it will appear on the Teen Health & Wellness Web site in "Dr. Jan's Corner."

If you have an urgent question on a health or wellness issue, we strongly encourage you to call a hotline to speak to a qualified professional or speak to a trusted adult, such as a parent, teacher, or guidance counselor. You can find hotlines listed in the For More Information section of this book, or at www.teenhealthandwellness.com/static/hotlines.

Some cells experience damage only to their outside layer, just as with bruising. In the case of cancer, damage to the outside layer or membrane of the cell does not lead to cancer. The kind of damage that a cell experiences from exposure to carcinogens, however, takes place inside the cell at its nucleus. Carcinogens can even damage or alter certain genes, leading to greater susceptibility to cancer.

Recent cancer research has discovered the existence of genes that may play a role in the development of cancer. Each human cell is controlled by more than thirty thousand genes. Genes can be understood as a set of instructions for the cells of the body. They determine much of our individuality. Our genes are inherited from our parents. We get one set of genes from our father and one set from our mother. The latest information on genes and cancer has led to the theory that cancer occurs when a series of altered or damaged genes accumulate or develop in a cell and begin sending out faulty instructions.

HOW ONCOGENES AND TUMOR SUPPRESSOR GENES WORK

It is likely that certain genes are responsible for predisposing an individual to cancer. There are genes called oncogenes, which appear to help cancer grow. On the other hand, another group of genes known as tumor suppressor genes seem to help slow or halt the growth of cancer.

Under typical circumstances, oncogenes play a normal role in cell growth. If the oncogene is altered in some way, however, perhaps due to exposure to a carcinogen, or if it appears in high levels, it may aid in the growth of tumors. Indeed, in some cases, oncogenes are normal genes that have been altered by exposure to carcinogens such as radiation and chemicals. In these cases, the oncogene can begin turning normal cells into tumor cells.

Genes instruct the cell in which they reside to maintain the cell's ordinary jobs, such as producing the

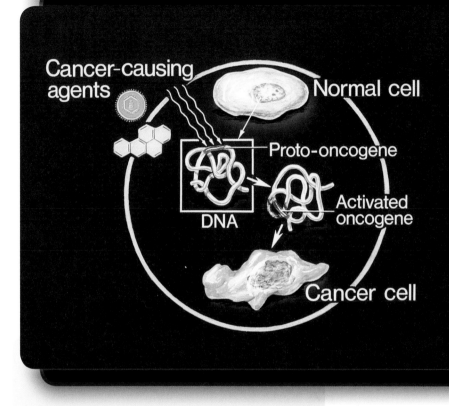

This graphic explains the process by which a normal, healthy cell becomes a cancerous cell once an oncogene becomes activated.

necessary amounts of proteins or chemicals. If the cell is exposed to radiation or certain carcinogenic chemicals, however, its DNA can be broken apart or otherwise altered. The separated or damaged DNA is then likely to reconnect incorrectly, forming an altered gene, or oncogene. Once the oncogene has been created and begins sending out its faulty instructions, the cell may produce unusually large amounts of one of its normal proteins or an altered protein. As a result, the cell alters its size, shape, and behavior. It has now become a cancer, or tumor, cell. Cancer cells look very different from normal cells.

When the cancer cell divides, each new cell possesses an identical copy of the problematic oncogene. This means the altered, tumor-promoting gene is already present in the new cells. When these new cells divide, they, too, pass on the same altered, tumor-promoting gene to the next generation of cells, and the process goes on and on. As this process of division continues, the rapidly reproducing cancer cells become a tumor. At this point, tumor suppressor genes attempt to do what their name implies: they try to stop cells from growing abnormally. In some cases, if the tumor suppressor genes are missing or damaged, a cell will continue to grow abnormally and make copies of itself without anything being able to stop it.

Damaged genes can be passed on within a family. If a person inherits the damaged genes, his or her chances of developing a certain kind of cancer are increased. If you know that some of your family members have been diagnosed with a certain type of cancer, you can speak with a genetic counselor. Genetic counselors can answer questions about specific genetic factors that may put you at risk for specific types of cancer. There are also tests that you can take for some kinds of hereditary cancers to determine if you were born with a higher risk of getting a specific disease because of your family history.

The following are some of the leading risk factors for many types of cancer:

- Unprotected exposure to strong sunlight or lengthy amounts of time in the sun
- Smoke from cigarettes (direct or secondhand)
- Chewing tobacco
- A high-fat, low-nutrient diet
- Excessive alcohol consumption
- Little or no physical activity
- An inherited predisposition to developing certain cancers
- Exposure to chemical solvents
- Exposure to radiation

If any of these risk factors apply to you, it should prompt you to make changes to your lifestyle that will result in lowering your cancer risk. It should also prompt you to schedule regular checkups with your doctor, who should be made aware of any relevant family and personal medical history and risk factors. Working toward better health and avoiding cancer risks are excellent and often very effective forms of cancer prevention.

WHAT ARE THE ODDS?
CANCER RISK FACTORS

Avoiding illness is all about avoiding or decreasing risk factors. Many risk factors can be easily avoided, such as smoking cigarettes or exposing oneself to harmful ultraviolet (UV) radiation without sunscreen. Certain

RISK AVOIDANCE

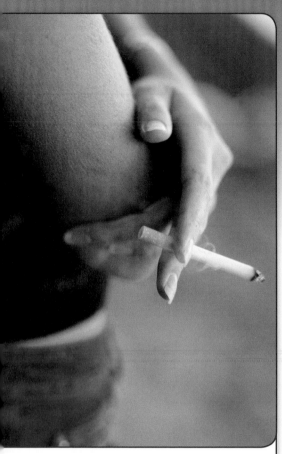

Cigarette smoking will greatly increase one's chances of developing any numbevr of cancers. Quitting smoking at any age greatly reduces the chances of developing cancer.

individual factors, or inherited risk factors, are unavoidable, however.

Inherited risk factors relate to the kind of cancers that exist in a family's history and if this history may put a person at increased risk for developing cancer. The chance of developing a cancer that runs in the family depends on what type of cancer it is. A medical family history can help a patient and physician identify that patient's unique risk factors for specific types of cancer. People who have an increased likelihood of getting cancer due to family history and genetics can help protect themselves by avoiding other risk factors for that cancer and by getting regular checkups. Only a few rare cancers are caused solely by heredity. Most have an environmental component—exposure to certain carcinogens like cigarette smoke, toxic chemicals, radiation, or the following of a poor diet.

Certain other diseases and infections can increase the risk of developing some types of cancer. For example, infection with the human papillomavirus (HPV) increases a woman's risk of developing cervical cancer. There are also some medications that increase the risk of developing cancer. Your doctor should be able to answer any questions you might have about the risk factors posed by your medications or previous and current illnesses.

CHAPTER 4

Many people have the idea that cancer is both an unpreventable and untreatable disease—a cruel stroke of fate about which nothing can be done. It is important to know, however, that there are many things that can be done to greatly reduce the likelihood of ever developing cancer. Consider some of the following statistics:

- According to the American Cancer Society's 2010 report on cancer facts and statistics, all cancers caused by cigarette smoking and the overconsumption of alcohol could be prevented completely.
- More than 170,000 cancer deaths annually in the United States are attributed to tobacco use.
- Each year, about 20,000 cancer deaths are related to excessive alcohol use, frequently in combination with tobacco use.
- About 3,400 nonsmokers die each year from lung cancer because of a spouse or family member who smokes. Secondhand smoke also causes the deaths of 46,000 nonsmokers due to heart disease.
- A nonsmoker married to a smoker has a 30 percent greater risk of developing lung cancer than a person who is married to a nonsmoker.
- Smokers are about ten times more likely to develop lung cancer than are nonsmokers. Tobacco smoke contains thousands of chemical

agents, including sixty known carcinogens. Secondhand smoke alone contains four thousand substances, fifty of which are considered cancer causing.

- Almost half of all smokers between the ages of thirty-five and sixty-nine die prematurely. Smokers could be losing an average of twenty to twenty-five years of their lives. People who quit smoking, at any age, live longer than those who continue to smoke. People who quit smoking before the age of fifty cut their chances of dying within the next fifteen years by half.

- Quitting smoking greatly reduces the risk of developing cancers of the lungs, pancreas, esophagus, larynx, mouth, bladder, and cervix, and lowers the risk for heart disease and stroke.

- One-third of the more than half million cancer deaths per year in the United States are related to being overweight or obese, physically inactive, and/or having a poor diet. These are highly preventable cancers and deaths.

- It is estimated that 50 to 75 percent of cancer deaths in the United States are caused by human behaviors such as smoking, lack of exercise, and poor dietary choices. Physical activity can actually lower the chances of developing some cancers (including colon cancer) by 50 percent.

- Cancers related to certain infections, such as hepatitis B, HPV, and HIV, can be prevented by lifestyle changes, antibiotics, and/or vaccinations.

- The more than one million skin cancer diagnoses made annually in the United States could be

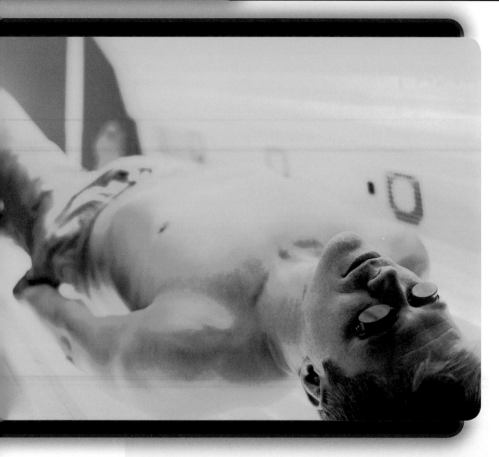

Exposure to ultraviolet (UV) radiation increases one's risk of developing skin cancer. Overexposure to UV rays also damages the skin and can lead to its premature aging and wrinkling.

prevented by avoiding or guarding against harmful sunlight, UV light, and indoor tanning.

- Regular checkups and screenings by medical professionals can detect precancerous growths and lead to their removal before cancer has a chance to develop and spread. This is particularly true of colon, cervical, and rectal cancer. Regular checkups and screenings can also result in early diagnosis of cancer, when the disease is most treatable and curable. This is particularly true of breast, colon, rectal, cervical, prostate, oral, and skin cancer. Cancers that can be prevented or detected early through regular checkups and screenings account for about half of all new cancer cases each year.

- More than 90 percent of all skin cancers develop on the face, neck, ears, forearms, and hands, which are all regularly exposed to UV rays. Many of these cancers can be prevented by avoiding the sun's harmful rays, using sunscreen, and avoiding indoor and outdoor tanning.

A FAMILY AFFAIR: PREVENTING CANCER

Knowing the risk factors, and avoiding the behaviors associated with those factors, can lower one's chances of developing cancer. This is the best kind of prevention. Often, a group effort is needed in order to reach the goal of cancer prevention and assure that every family member and loved one lowers his or her chances of developing it.

For example, a family member may drink alcohol and smoke. Obviously, the carcinogens in these substances can increase the user's risk of getting cancer. Smoking, in particular, also constitutes a risk factor for the rest of the

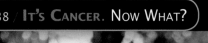

smoker's family through carcinogenic secondhand smoke. It is up to the other family members to point out the risks this person is running and urge him or her to avoid the bad habits that may literally kill him or her and negatively affect the health of everyone else around. If members of the family are interested in preventing cancer, the following guidelines can help them reach their goal of prevention.

NUTRITION AND PREVENTION

The American Cancer Society and the National Cancer Institute publish nutrition guidelines for dietary practices that reduce cancer risk. These guidelines are based on existing scientific evidence that connects diet and nutrition to cancer risk. Many dietary factors can affect cancer risk: types of food, food preparation methods, portion sizes, fat content, and food variety.

One of the best ways to prevent cancer through nutrition is to lower the consumption of fats. Certain kinds of fat are bad for the body because they can clog arteries and cause heart disease. The best kind of fat is polyunsaturated fat. Polyunsaturated fats don't raise the body's blood cholesterol level as do other fats, so they're better for one's health. They are found in many vegetable, sunflower, and soya oils (oils made from soybean products).

Eating more vegetables is one great way to help prevent cancer. It is a good idea to steam vegetables rather than grill them, however. Charred foods are carcinogenic, which means they can actually cause cancer.

ASK DR. JAN, PSYCHOLOGIST

First Name: John

Question:
My parents both smoke in the house. I'm worried that inhaling their secondhand smoke will one day give me cancer. How can I talk to them about my worries and ask them not to smoke in the house (or quit smoking altogether) without making them mad?

Answer:
You are correct in thinking that breathing secondhand smoke is unhealthy for you and others in your home. It is important for you to be able to speak to your parents about your concern for their health and your own, yet to do it in a way that will be productive and not make them mad. Consider the following strategy:

1. Do some research on the effects of cigarette smoking and secondhand smoke, noting some simple points that you may want to share.

2. Think about what you will say to your parents and how you can say it respectfully.

3. Wait for a positive moment, when everyone is in a fairly good mood and has the time to have an open discussion.

4. Speak in a sympathetic tone. For example: "I know that nicotine is one of the most addictive drugs on the planet

and quitting can be really hard, but I love you both and worry about your health."

5. Include information that you learned and your concerns about secondhand smoke and suggest that the family work on a strategy (if your parents continue to smoke) that will help protect you and others in the house.

6. Give your parents time to think about it before making any decisions, perhaps scheduling a future time to check back with them.

7. Thank them for allowing you to share your feelings and concerns.

While it's easier to shy away from difficult conversations, being prepared and speaking in a sympathetic and respectful manner can often lead to a positive result. Even if your parents make no changes, which hopefully they will, you will at least have had the opportunity to express your feelings, and that's really important, too.

Ask a Question

Do you have a question that you would like answered? E-mail your question to Dr. Jan at drjan@rosenpub.com. If your question is selected, it will appear on the Teen Health & Wellness Web site in "Dr. Jan's Corner."

If you have an urgent question on a health or wellness issue, we strongly encourage you to call a hotline to speak to a qualified professional or speak to a trusted adult, such as a parent, teacher, or guidance counselor. You can find hotlines listed in the For More Information section of this book, or at www.teenhealthandwellness.com/static/hotlines.

Lean proteins, such as chicken and fish, are preferable to fatty proteins like non-lean beef. In addition, a diet largely consisting of fruits and vegetables and foods that are made from whole grains and are high in fiber is believed by many medical researchers to help prevent cancer, though studies have been inconclusive thus far. Fiber is believed to have a cleansing effect on the digestive system, scrubbing it of cancer-causing toxins. It is best to avoid any packaged or processed foods. Instead consume as much whole food as possible, eaten raw or cooked by yourself at home, where you can control the amount of sugar, salt, and fat that are added.

Fruits and Vegetables

Fruits and vegetables are foods that can help increase the amount of vitamins and other nutrients in one's diet, boost fiber intake, and lower fat consumption. Many are high in fiber and low in fat. In addition, fruits and vegetables contain compounds that are believed to help prevent cancer. Use the following alphabetized list to remember the different fruits and vegetables that can be helpful in preventing cancer. By eating at least five servings of them a day, one can significantly lower the risk of developing several types of cancer.

A: apples, apricots, asparagus, avocado
B: bananas, beets, berries, bok choy, broccoli, brussels sprouts

C: cabbage, cantaloupe, carrots, cauliflower, citrus
fruits, cucumbers
E: eggplant
G: garlic, grapefruit, green peppers
K: kale, kiwi fruit, kumquats
M: mango, melons
O: okra, onions
P: papaya, parsley, peaches, pears, peas, peppers, pota-
toes, pumpkin
R: radishes, romaine lettuce, red leaf lettuce
S: soy products, soybeans, spinach, squash
T: tomatoes, turnip greens
Y: yams
Z: zucchini

BETTER CHOICES, BETTER HEALTH

The following foods should be eliminated from one's
diet or at least greatly reduced. Each of them has been
linked to prostate, colon, rectal, or stomach cancer:

- Fatty red meats (beef, lamb, venison)
- Charcoal-broiled or barbecued and well-done foods
  (charred foods are carcinogenic)
- Smoked or processed meats (such as ham, bacon,
  and sausage)
- Pickled vegetables
- Foods and beverages that contain nitrates (salami,
  pepperoni, hot dogs, bacon)
- Salt-cured foods (such as jerky)

CUT THAT FAT!

Here are some easy tips for reducing fat consumption, preventing disease, and promoting good heath.

- Eat less meat, poultry, and other animal products. Instead, eat more soy products, such as tofu.
- Eat skinless, white meat chicken or turkey, rather than dark meat.
- Eat only lean cuts of meat and fish and reduced-fat lunchmeats.
- Eat more grains, breads, and starches.
- Use skim milk, rather than whole milk.
- Choose low-fat dairy products.
- Snack on fresh fruit, dried fruit, vegetables (like carrot and celery sticks), small quantities of unroasted nuts, and yogurt.
- Limit consumption of baked goods, which are high in fatty oils.
- Use low-fat cooking methods, such as broiling, grilling (though don't char the food; charred food is carcinogenic), baking, steaming, poaching, and microwaving, rather than frying.

EXCESSIVE ALCOHOL CONSUMPTION AND CANCER

In recent years, researchers have discovered increasingly strong links between alcohol use and cancer. Heavy, long-term use of alcohol can damage the liver. This can lead to liver diseases, including cirrhosis (scarring of the liver) and hepatitis (inflammation of the liver), both potentially fatal illnesses. Alcohol is also a recognized cause of liver cancer, a type of cancer that has an extremely high death rate. Half of the people who die from liver cancer were heavy drinkers. Risks associated with alcohol consumption vary considerably by type of cancer. The strongest associations between alcohol and cancer are with cancers of the mouth, esophagus, larynx, throat, breast (in women), colon, rectum, and liver.

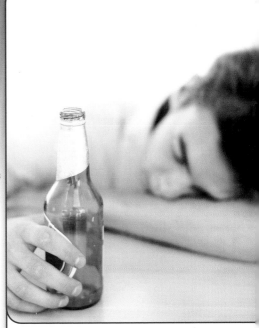

Overconsumption of alcohol is a leading cause of cancer, as well as other deadly diseases like cirrhosis of the liver.

Moderate alcohol use is key to the prevention of alcohol-related cancers. Many of the cancers related to alcohol result from heavy consumption, so reducing the level of alcohol consumption lowers the risk considerably. The American Cancer Society recommends that adults of legal drinking age should, in general, have no more than one alcoholic drink a day. Anyone who develops a dependency on, or an addiction to, alcohol should avoid it altogether, and anyone who has a family history of alcoholism should consider abstaining. Combining cigarette smoking with alcohol use enhances the cancer-causing effect.

Avoiding the Sun

Some people still believe that having a deep tan is a sign of good health and attractiveness, but a tan is actually evidence of damaged skin and greatly increased cancer risk. Sunlight contains ultraviolet rays, which can damage or even kill skin cells (in the case of severe burns). The damaged skin cells can eventually become cancerous.

Anyone going out in the sun—regardless of whether his or her skin is fair or dark—should use a sunscreen with a high SPF number. "SPF" stands for the "sun protection factor" that blocks both UVA (longwave) and UVB (shortwave) rays. The higher the SPF number, the more protected skin cells are from damage. For a good start toward skin cancer prevention, use a sunscreen with an SPF of at least 15. One can also decrease exposure to sunlight by wearing clothes that cover more skin (including a wide-brimmed hat) and avoiding sunlight from 10 AM to 4 PM.

In addition to seeing a dermatologist for a skin checkup every year, people should perform their own skin checks from time to time. These self-examinations can help you spot any odd changes to the skin, especially in moles or freckles. You should check yourself in a well-lit room just after taking a shower. Use mirrors for the parts of the body that cannot easily be seen. Get to know how the moles and birthmarks on your body look. As you check your skin from time to time, look for any changes, like a new mole or skin discoloration, or a sore that does not heal. Also look for any changes in the size, shape, texture, or color of existing moles. Anytime you see something different, let a parent or doctor know. Also, anything that you might apply to your skin, such as lotions and underarm deodorants, should contain natural products, rather than chemical mixtures. The skin can absorb the chemicals in these products and introduce them into the body's cells and bloodstream.

No Smoking!

The effects of smoking are responsible for most cancers of the larynx, oral cavity, and esophagus. In addition, smoking is strongly linked with the development of— and deaths from—bladder, kidney, pancreatic, and cervical cancer. Out of two thousand smokers under the age of eighteen, nearly seven hundred will die due to lung cancer or other tobacco-related diseases. We know that smoking is the direct and primary cause of some cancers and contributes to the risk of developing others.

Besides the fact that it contributes to a number of different cancers, smoking stinks! The clothes, hair, and breath of a smoker smell bad—and that's only what's happening outside the body. A smoker's teeth are often dull and yellow, and smoking ages the skin, leading to premature wrinkling. There is nothing fun about look-ing old when one is still young. Nicotine patches, gum, prescription drugs, and special counseling programs can help smokers who really wish to quit. There are no good excuses for smoking or for not quitting.

Get Moving!

Research has shown that gaining more than eleven pounds (five kilograms) in adulthood (after you are full grown) can increase the risk of cancer. Obesity has been linked to heart disease, diabetes, gall bladder disease, arthritis, and certain cancers, including colon and prostate cancer in men, and cervical, ovarian, and breast cancer in women. A person must try to stay within his or her healthy weight range, as determined by a doctor following an examination. The two best ways to avoid or combat obesity are to eat more healthfully and exercise more (always seek and receive a medical examination and a doctor's OK before beginning an exercise program).

If you do not get much exercise, become more active. If you are already very active, try to maintain the same level of activity as you age. You should try to do moderately active exercise for at least thirty minutes every day.

Minimizing Exposure to Radiation

X-rays release ionizing radiation, which is a known cause of cancer and has other adverse effects on health. This type of radiation changes the gene structures of the cells and damages them, making them more prone to cancerous growth. Avoiding unnecessary medical X-rays is one of the best ways to reduce exposure to ionizing radiation. In many cases, however, X-rays are absolutely

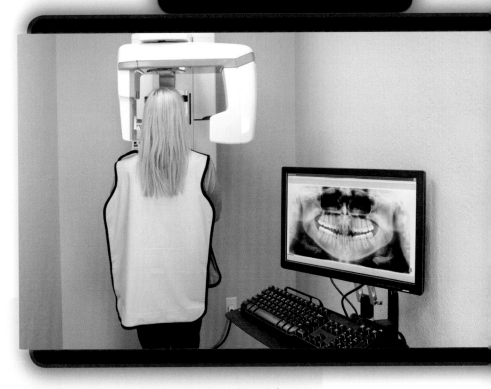

A patient wears a protective smock as she receives
a dental X-ray. While X-rays are important diagnostic tools, overexposure to them can cause cancer.

necessary for a doctor to make a diagnosis. To minimize
the patient's exposure to radiation, an X-ray technician
will place protective barriers on the parts of the body
not being X-rayed.

Some natural sources, such as elements and substances in Earth's crust, give off radiation. One substance
in particular, radon, has been linked to certain kinds of
cancer. Radon gas can seep up from the ground and into
homes. Houses can be tested for radon with test kits that
can be purchased at stores.

BETTER SAFE THAN SORRY: GO SEE THE DOCTOR

Annual checkups are essential for many reasons, one of the chief being cancer prevention or early diagnosis. If a doctor finds any development of cancer early, it can be treated before it spreads to other parts of the body. The earlier cancer is discovered, the better the patient's chances are for recovery and cure. If close relatives have developed cancer, it is important to let your doctor know and then follow his or her advice about cancer prevention and checkups to detect problems early.

For various reasons, the doctor's office is one of the last places many people want to visit. The main reason is that the doctor's office is associated with illness. After all, other than yearly checkups, most people see their doctors only when they are feeling poorly. Getting shots or having surgery at the hospital can be scary, too. But the truth is that visiting the doctor, getting shots, or having surgery is a necessary part of maintaining good health.

Doctors want us to be healthy. It is their job, their mission, and their passion. Being healthy is a lot more fun and life enriching than feeling sick and tired. And knowing what might keep a person and his or her body healthy is a lot better than not knowing. That's why it is important to think of visiting the doctor as a crucial part of getting better or maintaining good health by preventing illness.

Even when a person cannot see or feel their presence, growths inside the body often produce symptoms. Symptoms are what usually motivate a patient to see a doctor. They indicate that something is wrong within the body. For example, symptoms for the common cold are fever, aches, and coughs. Below is a list of symptoms that, besides being signs of more common and less serious illnesses, might also be signs of cancer. The important word is "might." People shouldn't immediately assume that they have cancer if they have some of the symptoms because, as said above, most of them are shared by many common illnesses. In any case, they do indicate that a person may need medical attention. If you are experiencing any of these symptoms, you should tell a parent or guardian and consult a doctor:

- Frequent infections
- A sore that does not heal
- Indigestion or difficulty swallowing
- Nagging cough or hoarseness
- Weakness and fatigue
- Loss of appetite and/or weight loss
- Easy bleeding or bruising
- Unusual bleeding or discharge
- Swollen or bleeding gums
- Swollen or tender lymph nodes
- Constant fever or chills
- Changes in bowel or bladder habits
- Obvious change in a wart or mole

If you notice any of these symptoms, it is important to tell a parent, guardian, or other responsible

REASONS TO SEE A DOCTOR

adult. Some things might seem embarrassing to say, for instance, "I keep having diarrhea," but you are responsible for your health. Anything that is bothering any part of your body affects your overall health. A person who is concerned about you will want to hear when things are not quite right. Again, these symptoms are not always a sign of cancer. They can also be caused by far less serious infections, benign tumors, or other illnesses. But no illness should be ignored.

If visits to the doctor's office still make you worry, do not keep these feelings to yourself. Tell your doctor or the medical staff how you feel. Talking to your doctor or nurse about your anxiety can help you relax.

DIY: Self-Examinations

Checking various parts of the body—such as the skin, lymph nodes, breasts, or testicles—for signs of tumors or other irregularities is an important aspect of health maintenance, cancer prevention, and early diagnosis. This is especially the case for female breast tissue, particularly if a woman has a family history of breast cancer. Women should check their breasts three days after their period ends (or on the same day every month if they do not menstruate regularly). The self-exam is easiest to perform in the shower. The pads of the fingers should be used to check both breasts for lumps. A woman should start with light pressure and then increase pressure until she gets a good feel for, and sense of, the breast tissue under the skin. The following areas of the breast should be checked:

- Outside: Armpit to collarbone, below the breast, and sides of body
- Middle: The breast itself
- Inside: The nipple area

The breasts should also be examined in a mirror to get a better sense of how they look. This will allow a woman to better notice any sudden changes to them. If a woman notices any liquid coming from the nipples, puckering of the skin, redness, or changes in the size or shape of the breast beyond normal growth during puberty, she should discuss this with a doctor and receive a medical examination. Many lumps and bumps develop in the breast and are not cancerous. Nevertheless, it's very important to have any lumps and bumps checked by a doctor.

CHAPTER 5

SCREENING AND TESTING FOR CANCER

Diagnosis is the identification of the presence of a specific disease or illness. Only a qualified doctor can make a diagnosis. A diagnosis is based on tests and a doctor's knowledge and experience. When making a diagnosis related to cancer, doctors take into account the patient's age, general health, medical history, family history, and lifestyle. If a patient has a sign or symptom that might indicate cancer, the doctor will do a physical exam and review that patient's medical and family history. Next, the doctor will either rule out the possibility of cancer or recommend more tests. The tests mentioned in this chapter are used differently depending on the individual situation.

Not all of the tests discussed here are necessary to diagnose every kind of cancer, and doctors know which ones are needed in order to find out about a specific suspected illness. The most commonly used tests include X-rays, biopsies, and laboratory tests of blood and urine. Some of the procedures are noninvasive and can hardly be felt. Others, however, involve going inside the body. Doctors realize that some test procedures can cause discomfort or pain. They do everything they can to minimize any discomfort or pain associated with some tests. If you feel any pain during a procedure, tell your doctor or nurse immediately. If you have fears and anxieties related to undergoing tests, that's normal. You should tell your nurse or doctor this so that he or she can show you how to lessen your anxiety before and during tests. Doctors and nurses are also very careful during diagnostic tests. This is because the results of the tests are accurate only if they are performed correctly.

VARIOUS KINDS OF CANCER TESTS

When blood is drawn to test for cancer, a physician or an assistant takes a small sample of it. The sample is sent to a lab where it can be analyzed. The presence of cancer in the body can cause blood loss, which may present itself as

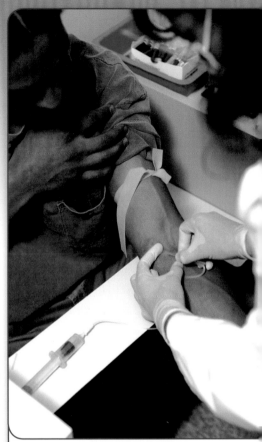

A nurse draws a patient's blood. Blood tests can be an important tool for detecting and diagnosing cancer.

anemia. Anemia means the red blood cell count is low, which the lab analysis will detect. Having anemia does not necessarily mean that a person has cancer, however.

When blood tests are used to look for abnormal levels of substances typically caused by the presence of cancer in the body, they are called markers. Two marker tests are CEA and PSA. CEA is the acronym for carcino-embryonic antigen, a substance produced by many types of cancer. PSA stands for prostate-specific antigen, which is produced when the male prostate becomes cancerous. Blood tests check for elevated levels of these antigens, which would indicate cancerous growth.

Urine tests can also be used to help determine the presence of cancer in the body. Doctors use a sample of the patient's urine to check for the presence of red blood cells, which can be a sign of illness.

A biopsy is the only sure way to diagnose a cancerous tumor. In a biopsy, the doctor removes a sample of tissue from the tumor or abnormal area. Sometimes, the entire tumor is removed. The tissue sample is looked at under a microscope to see if the cells are normal or cancerous. Biopsies can also show which type of cancer a person has and if the cells are likely to grow slowly or quickly. Biopsies are usually taken while the patient is under a local anesthetic (a numbing painkiller administered to the specific location being worked on), so he or she does not feel any discomfort or pain. A sample of tissue for a biopsy can be removed by surgery or by a needle, depending on the situation.

In another diagnostic method, the doctor examines the suspected cancerous areas while the patient is under a general anesthetic. A general anesthetic lessens sensation all over the body and sometimes results in the patient entering a deliberate state of sleeplike unconsciousness.

X-rays can also provide important clues about the presence or absence of tumors. If the results suggest the possibility of cancer, the doctor will probably recommend that the patient undergo a follow-up computed tomography (CT) scan (also referred to as a CAT scan). During a CT scan, the patient lies on a table that slowly slides into a large, tubelike machine. This scan is a type of X-ray that provides very detailed cross-section views of the inside of the body. It can show the exact location and size of tumors. It can also give clues as to the type of tumor and if the cancer is localized or has spread to other parts of the body.

Another type of scan is magnetic resonance imaging (MRI). MRI machines use large magnets and radio frequencies to produce highly intricate and accurate views of the inside of the body. The magnet is linked to a computer, which produces extremely detailed images that can be viewed onscreen and printed out.

An ultrasound diagnostic test uses high-frequency sound waves that cannot be heard by humans. These sound waves enter the body and bounce back to a receiver, where they are analyzed. The sound waves' echoes produce an image of the body's interior called a sonogram. The procedure is both painless and harmless. Ultrasounds can distinguish between tumors that are solid (more likely to be cancerous) and tumors that are filled with fluid (more likely to be benign). The resulting images are shown on a monitor and can be printed on paper.

An endoscopy is a diagnostic procedure that allows a doctor to look into the body through a thin, lighted, flexible tube called an endoscope. During the exam, the

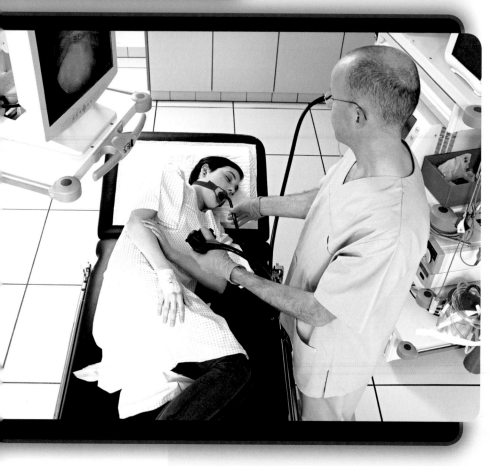

A young woman's esophagus is being examined by a doctor with the help of an endoscope.

doctor can collect tissue or cells that may look suspicious for closer study. When a specific organ is being examined, the exam is named for the organ. For example, a colonoscopy is an endoscopy performed inside the colon.

A bone marrow sample procedure is performed under a local anesthetic. Bone marrow is the soft, pulpy tissue found within some bones of the body. Tests of the marrow are ordered to determine if a cancer originating elsewhere in the body has spread to the marrow. Samples can also detect cancers of the blood and leukemias. A needle takes a sample of cells or tissue from the bone marrow, usually from the hipbone. The material obtained from the bone is examined under a microscope to determine whether it is cancerous or not.

A mammogram is a diagnostic test for breast cancer in women. The breast is placed between two plates that move closer together to compress the breast tissue, and an X-ray of the breast is taken. Being compressed in this way makes the interior of the breast easier to read on an X-ray. The doctor can see any breast lumps or growths on the resulting image.

A Pap smear test is a diagnostic procedure that is designed to detect cervical cancer. During a Pap test, samples of tissue are taken from the cervix. The doctor obtains the samples by gently using a small wooden spatula and a cotton swab to collect cells. The cells are analyzed for the presence of cancer.

Bone scans are designed to image only the bones, rather than the tissues that surround them. A small injection of a radioactive tracer substance is injected into the patient's arm vein. It travels through the bloodstream and is eventually absorbed by the bones. A special camera takes pictures of the tracer-infused bones. Any dark spots on the bones indicate the lack of absorption of the radioactive tracer and, therefore, a possible lack of blood supply to the bone or a certain type of bone cancer. Especially bright spots indicate areas that have

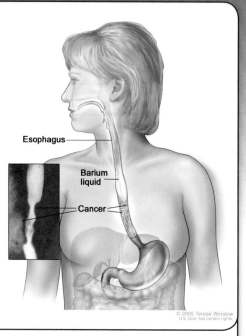

Esophagus

Barium liquid

Cancer

© 2005 Terese Winslow
U.S. Govt. has certain rights

This graphic shows how swallowed barium flows through the esophagus and into the stomach. When X-rays are taken, the barium highlights any abnormal areas.

absorbed greater amounts of the tracer, which may indicate the presence of a tumor.

Gallium scans focus on possible cancers of the lymphatic system. A small portion of a metal called gallium is injected into the body. Gallium shows up well on scans. It can give information about the status of any suspicious swollen lymph nodes. Similarly, barium is a metallic substance that shows up well on X-rays and helps highlight any abnormalities, such as polyps, tumors, ulcers, or enlarged veins. If a doctor is investigating the possibility of cancer of the stomach, esophagus, or digestive system, the patient will be asked to drink the barium, which travels through the digestive system. X-rays track the barium's journey, resulting in detailed images of the suspicious areas.

An EEG, or electroencephalogram, is an electrical recording of brain activity. Small recording devices are taped onto the scalp. They record the brain's processes while the patient's eyes are open, closed, and focused upon flashing lights. EEGs are used in diagnosing suspected tumors of the brain.

Doctors use several other kinds of tests in the diagnosis of cancer. Many of them are specifically designed for the diagnosis of a particular kind of cancer. Tests that are used for the diagnosis of cancer can also be used for preventative screening. Screening is checking for cancer, or conditions that can lead to cancer, in a person who does not yet display any symptoms. Routine screening tests are available for some types of cancer and can be done on a regular basis. Various screening tests may involve:

- Physical exams
- Lab tests
- Occult blood tests—the testing of stools (solid waste) for traces of blood, which may indicate colorectal or gastric cancer, polyps, or bleeding ulcers, among other conditions)
- Endoscopies
- Pap tests
- Mammographies

In recent years, an entirely new form of screening has emerged and is still being developed. This is genetic testing. It is designed to alert people to the likelihood that they will develop an inherited type of cancer, based upon a genetic tendency or mutation they may carry. This testing looks for certain gene mutations (changes) that are linked to some types of cancer. A person's DNA is analyzed to detect any genetic alterations that may indicate an increased risk for developing a specific disease or disorder.

OTHER DIAGNOSTIC TOOLS

The Importance of Routine and Preventative Screenings

Routine screenings, especially for those who are vulnerable to certain cancers either because of risk factors or family/genetic history, can help save lives and reduce suffering. This is especially true of cancers of the skin, mouth, breast, lung, stomach, liver, cervix, ovary, prostate, testis (testicle), colon, and rectum. The earlier cancer is detected, the better the prognosis. The prognosis is the likely outcome of the situation. Your doctor should be able to recommend any screenings that would be especially useful or relevant to you based upon your and your family's medical history, your lifestyle, and your known risk factors. Many hospitals and clinics offer free screenings. You can call a clinic or hospital in your community to get more information.

Besides preventive screenings, preventive surgery may be an option for those who have a very high inherited or genetic predisposition to developing certain cancers. An example would be if a person's chances of getting breast cancer were extremely high, the breasts could be removed as a preventative measure. This surgery option is radical and drastically invasive, so it should be considered only after a thorough medical evaluation and counseling. Scientists are also looking into methods of using vitamins and medications, known generally as chemoprevention, to lower a vulnerable patient's risk of developing a certain cancer to which he or she is genetically predisposed.

CHAPTER 6

When patients hear that the diagnosis is cancer, the initial response is often shock and fear. Many people go numb, feel terrified, or get angry. Cancer is a diagnosis that can also make people experience feelings of extreme anxiety or stubborn denial. It is definitely a diagnosis that changes the behavior of the person—and of his or her family—forever. People who have faced a cancer diagnosis say that the feelings of shock do not last very long. Most people are able to accept it after a few weeks, but those first few weeks can be a roller coaster of emotions for all of those involved. It is quite normal to feel shocked, angry, sad, lost, or frightened when given a diagnosis of cancer.

DEALING WITH EMOTIONAL OVERLOAD

The emotions experienced by a person newly diagnosed with cancer—fear, anger, denial, anxiety, helplessness, and depression—can be overwhelming. These feelings can also change quickly, often without prompting. Many people are not used to feeling even one of these feelings, let alone all of them virtually at once.

A cancer patient's loved ones feel as if they should say something to try to make him or her feel better. The best thing that can be done for

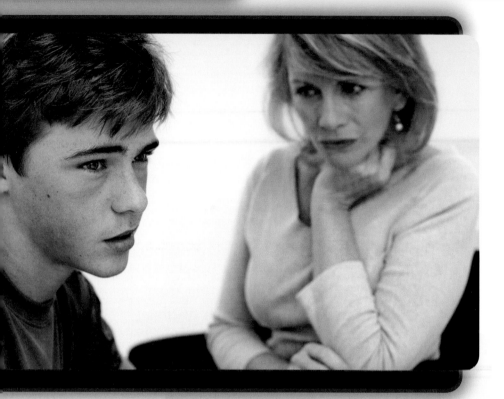

It is important to express your emotions honestly when dealing with cancer, even when those emotions may seem negative. Feeling anger, fear, sadness, and guilt are all perfectly normal when confronting cancer.

someone who is experiencing cancer is simply to listen. It might sound like such a small gesture in the face of the enormity of a cancer diagnosis, but letting someone express what he or she is feeling, at his or her own pace, is very helpful. All you need to do is show that you have all the time in the world to listen, that it is OK to say anything no matter how emotional, and that it is OK if the person isn't ready to talk yet.

If you have just received a diagnosis of cancer and are feeling any of the previously mentioned emotions, tell someone about it. If it is too difficult to talk to someone in your family, you can talk to counselors, nurses, social workers, psychologists, or spiritual leaders. The one emotion that you want to strive for while allowing yourself to feel all the other emotions swirling around you is hope. A diagnosis of cancer is neither a death sentence nor a hopeless situation. Prognosis and survival rates have improved greatly over the years for many types of cancers, and earlier and earlier detections have made the fight against cancer far more effective.

For most people, reaching a state of hope is the end result of an emotional process. The different stages of that process are discussed below.

"This Is Not True!": Denial

Denial is a refusal or inability to believe in the reality of a situation and make appropriate decisions accordingly. Denial is often one of the first responses to cancer. It sounds like a counterproductive reaction, yet denial serves a valuable protective function. It softens the impact of the diagnosis and allows a patient to adjust at his or her own pace. It becomes a problem, however, when the patient remains stuck in denial during the time when important and difficult decisions need to be made. While most patients work through their denial, there is counseling available for those who need help doing so.

ASK DR. JAN, PSYCHOLOGIST

First Name: Mary

Question:
There is a possibility that my cousin has cancer. She seems depressed, angry, and scared. It's hard to be around her right now. I feel terrible for her, but she is so angry and moody and negative and gets enraged anytime I try to talk to her about it. So I've been pulling away, which is probably the worst thing to do. I think she's in shock and really afraid of dying. How can I help her deal with the uncertainty of the diagnosis, the not knowing? How can I tell her that there may be nothing to worry about at all while also helping her to prepare for the worst?

Answer:
While we often hear about traumatic events happening to others, we rarely think that it will ever happen to us or someone we love. When it does, there is usually some initial level of disbelief. As you pointed out, your cousin probably is in shock, which would be a normal reaction to such overwhelming news. When we first hear that some-one we love is struggling, our initial reaction is to try and help. It may take a little while until your cousin is ready to deal with these feelings, which may be why she is reacting so negatively to your efforts to help. Consider simply letting your cousin know how much you love her and, if/when she wants to talk about her feelings, you are there for her.

It certainly is challenging for anyone to deal with an uncertain diagnosis of an illness that can be life threatening like cancer. In addition, most of us tend to deny our mortality because it is so overwhelming to consider. Unfortunately, your cousin is being forced to consider these really difficult issues, so it's not that surprising for her to be angry, moody, and negative right now. By letting her decide when and what she is ready to discuss, you will be able to fully support her by always being there to listen.

Ask a Question

Do you have a question that you would like answered? E-mail your question to Dr. Jan at drjan@rosenpub.com. If your question is selected, it will appear on the Teen Health & Wellness Web site in "Dr. Jan's Corner."

If you have an urgent question on a health or wellness issue, we strongly encourage you to call a hotline to speak to a qualified professional or speak to a trusted adult, such as a parent, teacher, or guidance counselor. You can find hotlines listed in the For More Information section of this book, or at www.teenhealthandwellness.com/static/hotlines.

"WHY ME?!": ANGER

Once a patient has accepted the diagnosis, he or she may experience anger. Many patients often ask, "Why me?" This is a perfectly normal and understandable question, but cancer is not personal. It doesn't deliberately and maliciously choose people to victimize. Anyone can get cancer. Good and bad people alike get cancer. People who carefully look after their health and do "all the right things" get cancer, while some lifelong smokers and heavy drinkers may not. Cancer is not a punishment, but it is a warning that you need to treat yourself the best that you can from here on out. Be kind to yourself, be healthy, and above all else, try to have hope.

Anger often arises out of feelings that are harder or less "acceptable" to express, such as fear, panic, and helplessness. Being angry can give a person the illusion of being more in control, more proactive and empowered, than do sadness, anxiety, and fear. If you or someone else in your family is experiencing anger, the best thing to do is to try to identify the reason. Any anger should be directed at the disease, not at the people around you. And the underlying fear and sadness that are giving rise to anger should be confronted and examined and, eventually, made peace with.

"WHAT IS GOING TO HAPPEN TO ME?": FEAR

Fears about cancer are based on the unknown. When a patient is diagnosed, fear can arise from concerns about pain, disfigurement, the side effects of treatment, medical bills and insurance, death, and so on. The best step to take toward conquering any fear is learning more about what scares you. Many patients have said that once they learned more about their kind of cancer, they were much less afraid. The loved ones of a patient feel fear because they worry that they will not be able to help enough or show enough love, that they won't be able to be there for the other person. Talk to someone if you are feeling fear about anything. Fear is a normal reaction, but it can be overcome by patience, open communication, knowledge, and hope.

"I'M FREAKING OUT!": STRESS

The uncertain time following a diagnosis of cancer can cause an enormous amount of stress that manifests itself in many ways. Stress can reveal itself physically by making the heart beat faster and by causing headaches, a loss of appetite, or dizziness. It also causes sleeplessness and nausea. Stress can weaken the immune system. These are things that the body does not need, especially while coping with a cancer diagnosis and treatment.

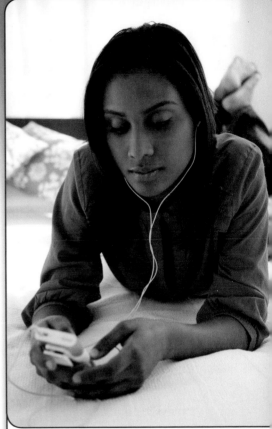

Taking time out to relax by listening to music, reading, or meditating can be an effective and health-giving stress-reduction strategy.

Action can be taken to lower stress levels. Patients have found physical, emotional, and mental relief from stress through deep breathing techniques, meditation, exercise, listening to music, reading a book, and talking about it to family members. A quick and easy way to get rid of some stress building up in your body and mind is to shake your arms and head and blow air through your mouth while saying, "Let it out," repeatedly, until the body feels loose and relaxed.

"I DON'T CARE ANYMORE": DEPRESSION

Some degree of depression is normal when a person is diagnosed with an illness such as cancer. Patients may experience despair and deep sadness. Depression becomes a problem when it lasts for an extended period or when the patient feels as if there is no longer any point to life. If you have experienced persistent feelings of despair and a lack of interest in your normal activities, and this mood has lasted for at least two weeks without change, tell your doctor. Depression can drain a person's energy, and energy is exactly what is needed most for cancer treatment. Your doctor can give you medication to help you through the depression and can help you get counseling.

"THIS IS ALL MY FAULT": GUILT

Family members of a cancer patient may feel guilty that they are in good health while their loved one is ill. They may also feel guilty because they feel there is little they can do to truly help the person with cancer. Cancer patients, in turn, may feel guilty because they think they have become a burden on the family. They may also feel guilty because they believe their own habits or behaviors contributed to the disease's development. There are support groups that can help everyone in a family deal with the feelings of guilt that arise along with cancer.

"I'm So Alone": Loneliness and Isolation

No matter how many people a cancer patient has around him or her, being diagnosed with the disease inevitably leads to profound feelings of loneliness. Some friends of the patient will not be able to handle the situation and may distance themselves. Physically, the cancer patient may tire easily and be unable to do all of the things that he or she is used to doing. The person with cancer may feel drained emotionally and not up to socializing, which is entirely understandable. A patient may also have to avoid public places that can be a source of infection. During treatment, extra care is taken to keep other illnesses from occurring in the patient. This can further isolate him or her from other people.

Treatment is a time to focus on getting better. However, feeling lonely and isolated can also weaken the immune system, which will not be helpful in fighting cancer. In order to fight feelings of loneliness, a patient can talk to other patients in support groups and even on the Web. It helps to know that others are going through the same things you are. You will also meet others during treatment. If a fellow cancer patient wants to talk, it may be a good opportunity to lessen your feelings of isolation and loneliness because he or she is going through the exact same thing. It may even give you an opportunity to express your fear, anxiety, anger, and sorrow and better come to terms with the disease.

"Things Are Good": Hope

A good dose of hope is the best emotional healer. There are excellent reasons to feel hope, even after a diagnosis of cancer. Modern treatment methods have helped millions of people become cancer survivors. They are now cancer-free. Other cancer patients are living many productive years with their cancer under control in the same way that people with other chronic diseases manage their illness. Because no doctor can predict with absolute certainty the course of the disease, there is always reason for hope, always. Some doctors believe that if a patient has a strong will to live and a positive attitude, it can make a difference in recovery. Talk with cancer survivors. They are a wonderful testament to the rich possibilities of life during and after cancer and the very real benefits of hope.

Talk It Out

Dealing with the emotions that accompany being diagnosed with cancer can help you deal more successfully with diagnosis, treatment, and life after cancer. Not every cancer patient reacts to life with cancer in the same way, but there is a coping method that has helped every person ever involved with cancer: talking about it. Talking about unpleasant thoughts and emotions is a good way to relieve the stress and suffering that they cause. Getting difficult issues out into the open is a positive experience because it releases the built-up tension that is caused by not talking about difficult issues. Anxieties that are suppressed fester and grow, often taking on a life of their own and growing out of proportion to the actual dangers of the situation. Speaking about one's worries and fears helps make them less dark and scary and robs them of much of their power and inflated size. Talking also allows the patient and those who care about the patient to operate on the same level of understanding and sensitivity about the situation.

There is often a time, in the days after the diagnosis, when cancer patients are not quite ready to discuss the situation. It is perfectly all right to say, "I don't feel like talking about it yet." The patient's loved ones should understand that discussion will occur when the time is right. Some loved ones may not be ready to talk about it when the patient is. Because of the difference in readiness for these conversations, it is hard to figure out the right time to share feelings about cancer. Because the people in our family know us so well, it sometimes takes an intimate expression to show that it's all right to talk, such as giving a hug and saying something like, "If you are worried, we can talk about it whenever you're ready."

SEEKING THE HELP OF MEDICAL AND COUNSELING PROFESSIONALS

There are many counselors who can help you understand, express, and cope with the emotions associated

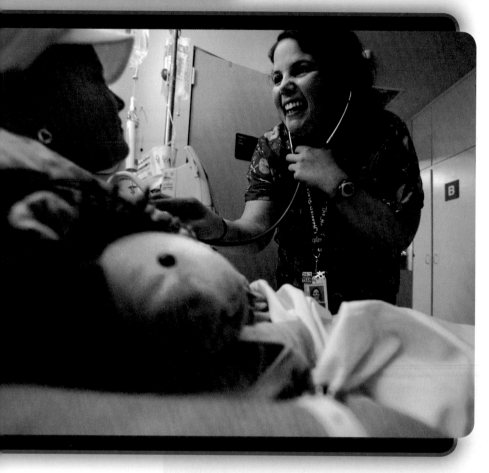

Pediatric oncology nurse and leukemia survivor Amanda Orlandella checks up on one of her young cancer patients.

with cancer. The different kinds of community counselors available to you are psychiatrists, psychologists, social workers, and religious representatives. Whom you decide to talk to is entirely up to you. You may also find that keeping a journal will help. You can write anything you want in it and look back on it later for reflection.

In order to most effectively guide your treatment and recovery, your doctor needs to know what you are really feeling, both physically and emotionally. Telling your doctor your feelings is not complaining, no matter how negative the feelings may seem. Open and honest communication with your doctor will reduce your anxiety and give him or her valuable information about your physical and emotional well-being that will help determine the course of care that he or she designs for you. Doctors' offices and hospitals may seem fast-paced and impersonal, but doctors and nurses are individually concerned with making each of their patients healthy and comfortable. Don't be afraid to speak up, ask questions, or tell a doctor that you need something.

Nurses are an extremely important part of your health care team. They are trained to be able to answer most of the questions you may have about your disease and its treatment. They can teach the family and the patient about ways to adapt to the changes in daily life that the disease and its treatment will create. Nurses are interested in your hopes, concerns, anxieties, and uncertainties as they relate to your health and sympathize with what you are experiencing. Nurses can also help you express your needs to the other members of the health care team— such as your doctors—and to your family and friends.

FINDING SUPPORT

Friends and family are crucial to the health and survival of people with cancer. A number of studies have linked cancer survival to social contacts. Being there for the patient, being a friend, is as easy as asking, "Is there anything you want to talk about?" Although the conversation does not have to be specifically about cancer, just the act of talking about other subjects will often lead to what is really uppermost in the person's mind. Or it will give the cancer patient a rare opportunity to talk about anything other than cancer, which is a blessing and a relief in itself. Also, patients will learn about their cancer at their own pace, so you don't have to worry about trying to educate them yourself. Just be there for them and let them set the pace and choose the conversational paths.

Talking with friends can help a cancer patient feel a lot better. When you talk with a friend about your concerns and fears, he or she can tell other people what kind of support or encouragement you need. Often, friends can comfort and reassure you in ways that others cannot. Getting the conversation started with them may be difficult. They are most likely scared that they will say or do the wrong thing. Many people do not yet understand cancer on a level that will allow them to cope, so they may withdraw from you. This gives you—as a patient or as someone who knows more about cancer—the opportunity to correct mistaken ideas. Once friends know that you are comfortable with talking about cancer, they will become more able to show support.

Sometimes, cancer patients need to speak to people who truly understand exactly what they are experiencing, both physically and emotionally. Friends try their best to understand and empathize, but if they are healthy, they can never truly appreciate your struggles. This is where support groups come in.

Support groups consist of people who are going through the same kinds of experiences you are. There are support groups to help cancer patients, some to help families of cancer patients, and others that help both. There is usually a leader of the group who helps guide the meetings. He or she may be a mental health professional (like a psychiatrist or psychologist) or a cancer survivor. At support group meetings, members can share their experiences, problems, concerns, feelings, hopes, and fears. The other members can offer information on how they dealt, or are dealing, with a similar situation. Members of support groups give each other encouragement, advice, emotional support, and positive energy. Support groups also work to educate patients or family members on advancements in cancer treatment and research.

Many people initially feel hesitant to join support groups. Some believe that it will be depressing or that people will say horrible things. The people who make the decision to go, however, are often very happy with the results and decide to attend more meetings. For cancer patients, support groups are beneficial because they can expand the patients' knowledge of cancer, reduce the feeling that they are alone in the fight, and increase their feelings of hope and purpose in life.

How to Be There for Someone with Cancer

There are some standard dos and don'ts when dealing with a person diagnosed with cancer. If you have cancer, you can share this list with people you love, which will help them understand your needs. If you know someone with cancer, the list can help you understand what his or her basic need are:

- Do not avoid the patient. He or she is the same person he or she was before the diagnosis, and you are the same person, too. Your relationship should not change because of the diagnosis.

- Do not be afraid to touch the patient or show warmth and love.

- Do not be afraid to laugh and cry with the patient. Allowing yourself to share in his or her feelings shows that you understand, care, and empathize.

- Never visit the patient without calling and getting permission first. There are days when any of us could do without seeing other people, and uninvited guests can be more work than fun. There is plenty of time to visit with the patient, so visit on the days that are best for him or her.

- Never visit the patient if you are feeling ill. Call instead. You don't want to expose him or her to additional illnesses.

- Don't feel as if you have to say something to make things better. Listening is far more important than talking.

- Don't be afraid to talk about life events that may occur in the future (going off to college, getting married, birth of children, a daughter's wedding, having grand-children, long-planned vacations, etc.) because you should assume that there is a future for the patient.

- Ask if you can help with the chores, and do as many as you can. The less that a patient has to worry about and expend energy on, the more he or she can con-centrate on getting better. If you are the patient, don't feel bad about asking someone to do something for you. You deserve a break.

- Send a card or call just to say, "Hello, I was thinking of you," or "I care," or "I am here for you." Little notes of love can go a long way.

- Focus on all of the positive things going on in the patient's life, rather than the negative things. It may be difficult to do, but positive energy can affect other people and the patient in a healing way.

- Tell the patient that he or she looks good. The patient might sometimes worry that he or she does not look as good as usual. If you are the patient, remember that treatment—and what happens to your appear-ance during it—is necessary for better health. If you lose your hair, weight, or general sense of self, you will get it back after treatment. Concentrate on getting better, not looking better.

Each support group is unique in its approach, number of members, and times that it meets. If you are fortunate enough to have a number of support groups to choose from, try to attend a few different meetings to find the right fit before deciding to become a regular member. You can find out about support groups in your area from your hospital's social services department.

RELAXATION TECHNIQUES

If you have cancer, there will be times when the only person who can help you is you. Only you can manage your stress. Remember that stress can have a negative impact upon your already fragile health. The best way to manage stress is to learn various relaxation techniques. There are a number of methods you can use to help yourself relax when dealing with cancer.

Visualization can help relieve stress and increase your sense of control. You can practice visualization anytime that you have a moment to concentrate. It works best when you can close your eyes and mentally remove yourself from distracting surroundings or noises. Try to create a detailed picture in your mind of what is going on inside your body as it is fighting, and winning, the battle with cancer. For example, some patients create a picture of armies of white blood cells attacking cancer cells, or they create a mental image of their cells being clean, perfect, and healthy. In moments when you feel pressured or overwhelmed, you can focus on this mental picture, which should relax and comfort you. You can also do this when you are already relaxed as a way of better connecting and harmonizing your mind and your body.

You can also visualize a place that is safe and comforting for you. Close your eyes and feel the muscles of your body relax. Then think of a place or scene that is comfortable and calm. Pretend that you are in that place. Perhaps it's the favorite room of your house, or a wildflower meadow on a sunny day, or the porch of a house on the beach.

Distractions are usually thought of as something negative, but distractions can actually be an aid in your fight against illness. In this sense, distraction consists of letting something—it can be just about anything—take your mind off what is bothering you. Examples of distractions are watching television or going to the movies, listening to music, and reading. There are distractions that can lead to self-discovery, such as doing something that you have always wanted to do but for various reasons have not yet explored. Examples of these kinds of distractions are learning to play an instrument, taking painting classes, learning to sail, or studying a new language.

Muscle tension and release is a relaxation technique that allows all the muscles in the body to relax. To start, lie down on a flat surface in a quiet room. Establish a slow, relaxed breathing pattern. Take a slow, deep breath, and as you breathe in, tense a particular muscle or group of muscles. Sometimes, it helps to start at the feet or the head.

For example, you can squeeze your eyes shut and scrunch your face with the muscles of the lips and jaw. At the end of the slow, deep breath, remain still for a second with the muscles tensed. As you breathe out, release the tension, and let the muscles relax completely. You can repeat this process until you have tensed and relaxed all of the muscles in your body.

Choosing a Medical Team and Designing a Treatment Plan

Following a diagnosis of cancer and after beginning the process of coming to terms with it, you should learn as much about your particular disease and its various treatment strategies as you can. This is still a time of personal crisis, which means you might not be able to correctly remember or interpret all the information you gather. Taking a friend or loved one along to doctor's appointments and consultations can help you better understand and remember the information. You can also compose a list of questions and give a copy to your doctor. This will allow him or her to answer your questions thoroughly, without getting sidetracked or interrupted. You can also ask permission to tape the discussion so that you can listen to it again later at home.

You will be seeing your doctor often, so there will be other opportunities to ask for more information. No question is foolish or inappropriate. Also, feel comfortable with asking a question more than once. If an answer to any of your questions is unclear, ask the doctor to explain it in a less complicated way. Here are some questions that a patient should ask the doctor:

- What is my diagnosis?
- What is the stage of the cancer?
- Is it a slow- or fast-growing cancer?
- Will the disease or its treatment affect my normal activities, such as school or work?
- Where can I learn more about this cancer?

Without answers to these questions, you cannot get an accurate understanding about the kind of cancer you have and what lies ahead. While researching your cancer, use only up-to-date and reliable information sources. Reliable information sources are cancer organizations (like the American Cancer Society and the National Cancer Institute), university hospital Web sites (like Johns Hopkins, Sloan-Kettering, and the Mayo Clinic), reputable medical Web sites (like WebMD), and library resources. Also remember that your case is unique, with its own individual prognosis and treatment plan. So whatever you read may not exactly mirror your cancer, symptoms, treatment, or experience.

Patients can also seek and receive a second opinion from another doctor. This is often advisable because it can reinforce the first diagnosis and treatment plan or offer you alternatives. This is standard practice and does not offend your doctor or imply doubt about his or her skills. It is just prudent to seek confirmation of a diagnosis and be aware of your range of treatment options.

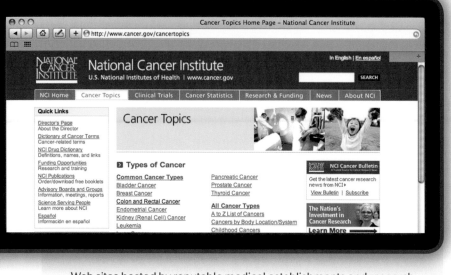

Web sites hosted by reputable medical establishments and research centers, like the National Cancer Institute (http://www.cancer.gov), can be excellent sources of information on the latest developments in cancer research, clinical trials, and treatment methods.

In general, if you are completely satisfied with the first doctor or specialist you consult, you do not have to get a second opinion, although it is highly recommended. A satisfactory doctor should be someone who listens to you and takes his or her time with you. Also, your doctor should be an effective communicator who cares that you understand what he or she is saying. You can ask if your doctor is board-certified in a particular specialty. He or she should also know of a good information network for you, which should include access to pamphlets, books, videos, support groups, or counselors. Most important, there should be a positive and creative energy between the two of you, which is an important part of the treatment and healing process.

The National Cancer Institute (NCI) provides a list of questions that can help you better understand the treatment that your doctor or team of doctors has planned for you. Some of the most important are:

1. Is the goal of this treatment curative (meant to bring about a cure) or palliative (meant to relieve symptoms only for a time)?

2. Why do you think this is the best treatment for me?

3. Is this the standard treatment for my type of cancer?

4. How safe is this treatment?

5. Are there other treatments?

6. Where is the best place to receive treatment?

7. Are there side effects with this treatment?

8. How can the side effects be relieved?

9. How will I know if the treatment is working?

10. Am I eligible for any clinical trials?

10 GREAT QUESTIONS TO ASK YOUR MEDICAL TEAM

There are numerous ways to treat cancer. The treatment strategy depends on the kind of cancer, its size and location, how advanced it is and if it has spread, the patient's age and general health, and other considerations.

CANCER STAGING AND GRADING

The stage of cancer describes how extensive the original (primary) tumor is and how far the cancer has spread in the body. If the doctor cannot tell immediately, he or she will most likely order tests in order to determine the stage of the cancer. In some cases, lymph nodes near the tumor can be removed and checked for cancer cells. If cancer cells are found in the lymph nodes, it may indicate that the cancer has metastasized, or entered the bloodstream and spread to other parts of the body.

There is no single staging system for all cancers. Some systems cover many types of cancer; others focus only on a particular type. The elements common to most staging systems, however, are the location of the primary tumor, the tumor size and number of tumors, the spread of cancer into lymph nodes, cell type, tumor grade (how closely the cancer cells resemble normal tissue), and the presence or absence of metastasis. One of the most common cancer grading systems, known as the TNM system, is based on the extent of the tumor (T), the extent of spread to the lymph nodes (N), and the presence of metastasis (M). A number is added to each letter (usually I–IV) to indicate the size or extent of the tumor and the extent of spread.

Three common terms that describe how far and to what organs the cancer has spread are "in situ," "invasive," and "metastasized":

- In situ cancer is confined to the place where it started. It has not spread.
- Invasive cancer is cancer that has spread from the tumor to nearby and surrounding tissues.
- Metastasized cancer is cancer that has spread to other parts of the body.

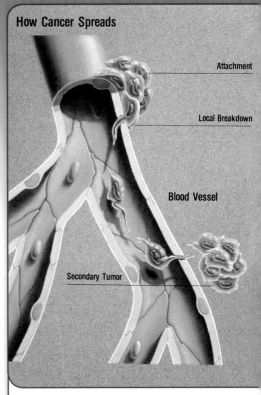

How Cancer Spreads

Attachment

Local Breakdown

Blood Vessel

Secondary Tumor

This graphic explains metastasis, the spread of cancer beyond its original location. Metastatic cancer cells enter the bloodstream, forming a secondary tumor elsewhere in the body.

The grade of a cancer is essentially a prediction regarding whether the cancer cells will grow quickly or slowly. To determine the grade, tumor cells are examined under a microscope in a lab to see how much they resemble normal, healthy cells. A doctor called a pathologist will be able to predict the growth rate of the cancer cells following this close observation.

Treatments that work for one patient may not be right for another, even if both patients have the same kind of cancer at the same stage. The results of treatment also vary in each particular case. The choice of treatment depends on the type and location of the cancer, the stage of the disease, the patient's age, and the patient's general health.

The Medical Team

Patients with cancer are often treated by a team of doctors who are specialists. These are physicians who have highly specific training in a particular area of medicine. Specialists in cancer care include the following:

- Hematologist: A doctor who specializes in blood diseases.
- Oncologist: A doctor who specializes in treating cancer.
- Pathologist: A doctor who specializes in the study of cells and tissues removed from the body (biopsy and surgery).
- Radiation oncologist: A doctor who specializes in using radiation to treat cancer.
- Radiologist: A doctor who specializes in the making of images of areas inside the body. The images are

made with X-rays, sound waves, and other types of energy. Radiologists can also explain and interpret the information that comes from the images.

THE FOUR MOST COMMON TYPES OF CANCER TREATMENT

There are four main types of cancer treatment, and there are other kinds of treatment that can be used in combination with these four main types. The treatments aim to destroy cancer cells and bring about what is called a remission. Remission means that through treatment, the cancer cells and symptoms disappear. When this happens, the cancer is said to be "in remission." Being in remission is not the same thing as being cured. After the goal of bringing about a remission has been accomplished, doctors work on maintaining the remission and curing the patient entirely of the cancer. A remission can last for months or years. If it lasts long enough, the patient is considered cured. The time it takes to be considered cured varies for different cancers. For many types of cancer, a patient is considered cured after being in remission for five years.

Depending on the type of cancer that is diagnosed, either a single kind of treatment or therapy or a combination of treatments can be used. Treatments can either target the whole body or specific areas. Local treatment attacks cancer cells only in one area, rather than treating healthy and unhealthy cells throughout the entire body.

Before starting any cancer treatment, you should give your doctor a list of any and all medications or vitamins that you take. The list should include descriptions of the medications, including how often you take them, the reason why they are needed, and their dosages. You also need to ask your doctor which kind of pain relievers you are permitted to take before, during, and after the treatment period. Once your treatment begins, always check with your doctor before taking any new medicines.

The four main types of treatment for cancer are surgery, radiation therapy, chemotherapy, and biological therapy. The other kinds of therapy that can be used in combination with these four main types of treatment are bone marrow transplantation, adjunctive therapy, and hormone therapy. Be sure to ask your doctor or nurse for pamphlets that describe the treatment that is being administered. You need to learn about and anticipate certain symptoms that can occur during the treatment. There are also certain physical activities you can perform or foods you can eat to make the treatment easier on your body. Similarly, certain other activities and foods should be avoided because they may make you feel worse during treatment.

Surgery: Removing the Tumor

Surgery is a cancer treatment strategy used to remove a tumor from the body. It is used for cancers that have a low tendency to spread. During surgery, all of the cancerous tumor or part of the tumor is cut out. Tissues

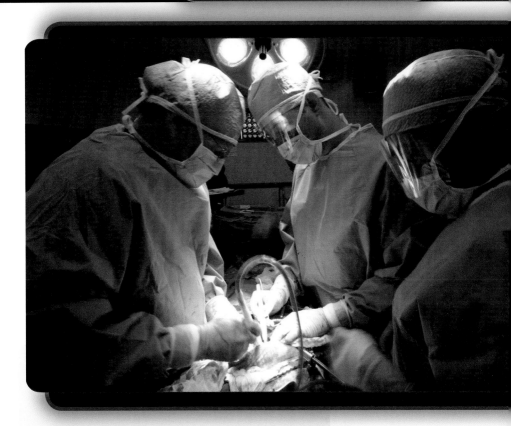

Surgeons perform surgery to remove four metastatic tumors from a patient's liver. The patient's original cancer was in the colon.

around the tumor and nearby lymph nodes may also be removed. For many solid tumors, surgery is the primary and most effective cancer treatment. A patient may receive radiation before the surgery in order to make the tumor smaller or make the surgery safer for the patient.

Tours of the operating room and recovery rooms can be arranged for patients who are anxious or fearful about the surgery. Visiting these places can bring about a feeling of familiarity that can replace fear, especially of the unknown.

Doctors should discuss with patients the possible side effects of having surgery. The side effects of surgery depend on the type of operation that is performed. Other factors that influence possible side effects are the patient's general health and the location of the tumor. Some patients experience discomfort or pain for a few days after surgery. Those patients are given medications to relieve their discomfort. Most surgeries require a stay in the hospital, but some can be performed on an outpatient basis (the patient does not have to spend the night at the hospital but simply visits the hospital, clinic, or doctor's office for the procedure and leaves soon after).

After surgery, it is common for patients to feel weak or tired for a while. There may be some activities that they should avoid until they have fully recovered from the surgery, such as heavy exercise, climbing stairs, or lifting heavy objects. The length of time it takes to recover from surgery is different for each patient, but the side effects (besides scars) are not permanent. There are some questions specific to surgery that you can ask your doctor:

- What type of anesthetic (numbing substance) will be used?
- What are the likely side effects of the surgery, and how can they be relieved?
- How long will I have to rest after surgery?

One alternative to traditional surgery that has emerged in recent years is cryosurgery—the freezing and killing of abnormal and cancerous cells. It can be used for external tumors, like skin cancer, or internally for certain kinds of liver, prostate, cervical, retinal, and bone tumors.

In some cases, another alternative is laser therapy. Some tumors can be shrunk or killed when bombarded with a high-intensity, focused beam of light. Laser therapy is especially useful in treating superficial cancers (on the surface of the body or the lining of organs), like skin cancer, and in the very early stages of certain cancers (cervical, penile, vaginal, and some lung cancers). Sometimes, the lasers are used in conjunction with photosensitizing agents that are injected into the patient's bloodstream and absorbed by the body's cells. The photosensitizer that is present in the cancer cells will absorb the laser's light and produce a form of oxygen that will destroy all nearby cancer cells.

RADIATION: ATTACKING CANCEROUS CELLS

Radiation therapy has been used for more than one hundred years in the treatment of cancer. Radiation therapy, or radiotherapy for short, uses high-energy rays aimed at cancer cells to kill or damage their DNA in order to prevent them from continuing to grow and divide out of control. The radiated cancer cells die because they

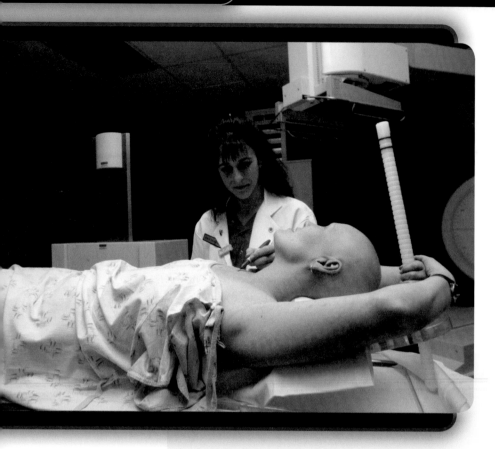

A medical technician prepares a woman for radiation therapy to treat breast cancer.

are so damaged that they can no longer divide. Normal, healthy cells close to the tumor are also damaged, however, which can cause illness in the patient.

Radiation therapy is usually given on an outpatient basis in a hospital or clinic five days a week for several weeks. The actual treatments may take only a few minutes each time. The amount of high-energy rays used will depend on the individual patient. To make sure that the rays are aimed correctly and the dosage is appropriate, high-tech scanners are used to create an image of the tumor before each session. This allows doctors to gauge the tumor's current size and location. Then computer programs calculate the required number of beams and angles of the radiation treatment.

Recently, the U.S. Food and Drug Administration (FDA) has approved proton therapy for use as an additional radiation therapy. Unlike high-energy X-rays, which have no charge, protons deliver a positive, deep, and very precise beam, causing more damage to the targeted tumor and less damage to surrounding healthy cells.

Using high-energy beams delivered by a machine outside the body to shrink tumors is known as external-beam radiation therapy. Yet in some cases, radiation can be administered by surgically inserting radiation implants (known as pellets or seeds) into the tumor. This is called internal radiation therapy, or brachytherapy. Internal radiation therapy can also be administered in pill or injection form. The patient stays in the hospital for a few days and the implant may be temporary or permanent. Some patients get both external and internal radiation therapy. About half of all patients receive some kind of radiation therapy at some point during their treatment for cancer.

The side effects of radiotherapy depend on the part of the body that is treated and the dosage. Some typical side effects are weakness, loss of appetite, and rashes or redness on the skin of the treated areas. Treatment may also cause a decrease in the number of white blood cells, which help protect the body against infection. This means the patient can get sick more easily, so precautions against exposing the patient to germs and viruses must be taken. Although the side effects of radiotherapy can be unpleasant, the doctor can usually treat or control them. In most cases, they are not permanent. The questions that you should ask your doctor about radiation are:

- What type of radiation therapy will I be getting?
- How long do the treatments take, and how many will I need?
- What do I do if I have to miss a treatment?
- What side effects should I expect after radiation?
- Do I have to change what I eat and drink?
- What can and can't I do physically during, after, and between treatments?

CHEMOTHERAPY: USING CHEMICALS TO FIGHT CANCER

Chemotherapy uses chemicals and drugs to destroy cancer cells. The use of chemotherapy started in the 1940s, when it was discovered that cancer cells became vulnerable when exposed to drug and chemical compounds. Depending on the type of cancer and its stage, chemotherapy can be used to cure cancer, slow or stop the cancer from spreading, or kill cancer cells that may have spread from the primary tumor to other parts of the body.

Because some drugs work better together than alone, chemotherapy may consist of more than one drug. This is called combination chemotherapy. How often and how long a patient receives chemotherapy depends on the kind of cancer, the goals of the treatment, the drugs used, and the body's response to the treatment. Chemotherapy may be used every day, every week, or every month. It is given in cycles that include rest periods so that the body has a chance to regain the strength that is sapped by the treatment and build healthy new cells. Chemotherapy attacks both healthy and cancerous cells, often causing weakness and illness in the patient, so this recovery period is crucial to the treatment's success. Your doctor should be able to estimate how long and how often you will be getting chemotherapy.

The chemicals or drugs are usually injected into the bloodstream and distributed throughout the body, attacking cancer cells anywhere they are growing. Chemotherapy can also be administered orally (by mouth) in pill or liquid form. It can also be applied topically (onto the skin). When chemotherapy is administered via needle, it can be injected into a muscle, an artery, or a vein (intravenously).

When chemotherapy is given using an intravenous needle (IV), the chemicals drip down from a bag through a tube that connects to the needle. The patient will sit or recline in a comfortable position and remain still while the chemicals are passing from the needle into a vein in the body. When an IV is started, some patients feel coolness or other unusual sensations in

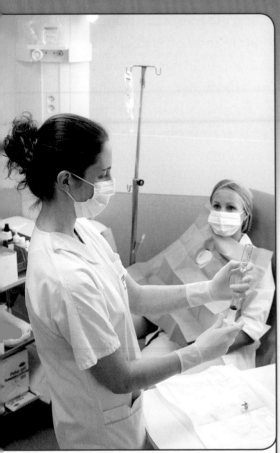

A nurse attends a woman receiving chemotherapy. Because chemotherapy can destroy healthy white blood cells, infections are common, so masks must be worn during treatment.

the area of the injection. It is important for patients to report any pain, burning, or discomfort that occurs during or after an IV treatment.

Usually, patients have chemotherapy on an outpatient basis, meaning they go home soon after the treatment has ended without having to stay overnight. Outpatient treatments can be administered at the hospital, at the doctor's office, or even at home. Where you receive treatment depends on the kind of chemo that you are getting, the hospital's policies, and your doctor's preferences. Patients should never miss a treatment, since it might interfere with the effectiveness of the treatments they've already received.

Whether or not a patient experiences certain side effects depends on the kind of chemotherapy used and how the body reacts to it. Every patient does not experience the same side effects, and some patients experience few, if any. The side effects of chemotherapy can include nausea, vomiting, hair loss (alopecia), and fatigue. Other side effects can include an increased chance of bleeding, infection, or anemia (low red blood cell count). Such side effects occur because, in addition to attacking cancer cells, chemotherapy also affects normal, healthy cells. Most normal cells recover quickly when chemotherapy is over, so most side effects gradually go away after treatment is stopped.

The time it takes to get over any side effects and regain energy varies from patient to patient. How soon you will feel better depends on your overall health and the kinds of chemotherapy drugs you are taking. Patients receiving chemotherapy can sometimes become discouraged by how long the treatment is taking and the side effects it may produce. If this happens to you or someone you know, talk to your doctor. Doctors may be able to suggest ways to reduce the side effects or make them easier to handle.

One of the largest concerns about side effects is that chemotherapy can make a patient very susceptible to infections. This is because infection-fighting cells (the white blood cells of the immune system) are killed along with cancerous cells during treatment. An infection can begin in almost any part of the body, including the mouth, skin, and lungs. Your doctor will check your blood cell count often while you are receiving treatment to make sure your immune system isn't becoming too weak or compromised. He or she may also decide to give you a series of shots that help boost the immune system. Some patients experience pain or aches in the bones after receiving these shots. This pain will subside after the series of shots is through. If your white blood cell count is still low after these shots, your doctor may postpone further chemotherapy treatments or lower the dose of the chemo for a while.

Questions to ask your doctor about chemotherapy are:

- Which drugs are you using for the treatment?
- What side effects can I expect from these drugs, and how can I relieve them?
- Are the side effects permanent or temporary?
- Where and how will I be receiving the treatment?
- Do I need to follow a special diet before, during, or after treatment?

Biological Therapy: Spurring the Immune System into Action

Biological therapy, also known as immunotherapy, is a treatment that uses the body's own immune system to attack cancer. It uses substances to try to boost the immune system's ability to fight infection and disease, including cancer. Biological therapy can also be used to protect the body from some of the side effects experienced as a result of other cancer treatments.

The substances used most commonly in biological therapy are monoclonal antibodies, interferon, interleukin, and colony-stimulating factors. The doctor will choose the substances to be used based on your specific medical situation. In addition, much research is being conducted on vaccines to protect against the development of certain kinds of cancers, including cervical lymphoma, melanoma, leukemia, and cancers of the cervix, brain, breast, lung, kidney, liver, ovary, prostate, pancreas, colon, and rectum.

The side effects of biological therapy depend on the type of treatment used and the individual patient. The side effects can include flu-like symptoms such as chills, fever, weakness, loss of appetite, nausea, vomiting, muscle aches, and diarrhea. Other possible side effects are rashes, bleeding, and easy bruising. Therapy that uses interleukin can cause swelling. If the side effects are severe, patients may need to stay in the hospital during treatment. They are usually not permanent and disappear once treatment has stopped. Some questions to ask your doctor about biological therapy are:

- What therapy will I be given, and how will it be given to me?
- Will I need to follow a special diet during treatments?
- How long will the treatments last?
- Will I have to stay in the hospital?

One new exciting area of research in this field is gene therapy. Medical researchers are exploring ways to use patients' own genetic material—their DNA and RNA— to fight cancer in various ways. Some experiments involve the replacement of missing or altered genes that may cause cancer with genes that are healthy. In other experiments, gene therapy is being used to improve the body's immune system response to cancer.

One of these methods is the injection of certain genes into white blood cells extracted from and re-injected into the patient. These genes instruct the white blood cells to produce T cell receptors, which direct the white blood cells to attacks tumors. Other experimental gene therapies involve efforts to make cells more sensitive to chemotherapy and radiation, while also making them more resistant to the side effects typical of those treatments. There is even research devoted to "suicide genes" that, once injected into cancer cells, will instruct those cells to destroy themselves.

BONE MARROW TRANSPLANTATION: PRODUCING HEALTHY BLOOD CELLS

Some cancer treatments destroy healthy bone marrow when they are administered in high doses. Since bone marrow is needed to produce blood cells, it is important to maintain its health. Bone marrow contains immature hematopoietic (blood-forming) stem cells that eventually develop into white blood cells that fight infection, red blood cells that carry oxygen, and platelets that help blood to clot. Bone marrow transplantation is the medical procedure that extracts healthy marrow from a donor, harvests stem cells,

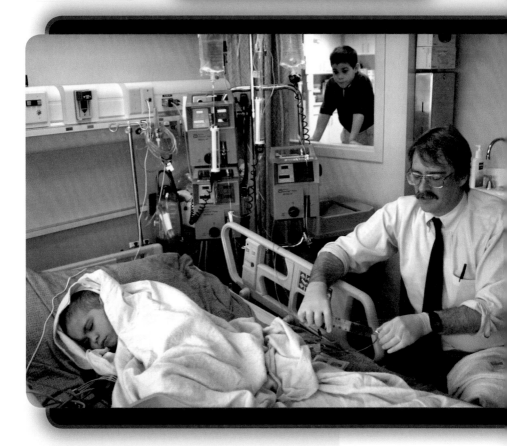

A young boy with leukemia receives a bone marrow transplant. The marrow was provided by his brother, visible in the background.

and injects them into the vein of the patient who has received a dangerously high dose of cancer treatment, such as chemotherapy or radiation. The donor can be a sibling, a parent, or even the patient (one's own stem cells can be harvested in some cases). A nonrelative who happens to be a good genetic match can also be a bone marrow donor.

A syringe inserted into the pelvis is used to take marrow from the donor. The cancer patient is given a strong dose of radiation and/or chemotherapy and, after a period of time, is injected with the new marrow. If the bone marrow transplantation is successful, the patient is able to receive very high doses of chemotherapy and/or radiation, increasing his or her chances of killing the cancer.

Some questions to ask your doctor about bone marrow transplantation are:

- What are the risks involved?
- Will I need to follow a special diet before, during, or after treatment and transplantation?
- Where will I receive the treatment and transplantation?
- How will I know if the transplantation was successful? How soon will I know?

ADJUNCTIVE THERAPY: IMPROVING THE ODDS

Doctors also use what is called adjunctive therapy. Adjunctive therapy is when an additional form of therapy, such as radiation, is used after surgery to reduce the chance that the cancer will come back. At the time that adjunctive therapy is administered, the patient is considered to be cancer-free. The additional therapy decreases the risk that the cancer will come back. The questions that you should ask your doctor about adjunctive therapy are:

- What kind of adjunctive therapy will I receive, and how is it given?
- Has this kind of therapy been proven effective against my type of cancer?
- Will I need to change what I eat and drink?
- What are the expected side effects, and how can I relieve them?
- Where will I be receiving adjunctive therapy and for how long??

One interesting and promising new type of adjunctive therapy is hyperthermia. It is used in conjunction with chemotherapy and/or radiation. Hyperthermia simply involves heating the body tissue containing cancerous cells to about 113 degrees Fahrenheit (45 degrees Celsius). High temperatures seem to damage and kill cancer cells without harming the surrounding healthy tissue. Hyperthermia also seems to make cancer cells more vulnerable to radiation and certain anticancer drugs.

HORMONE THERAPY: INHIBITING TUMOR GROWTH

Some types of cancer, including most breast and prostate cancers, need certain hormones to grow. Hormone therapy keeps these hormones from reaching the cancer, blocking its "food supply." Sometimes, the patient has surgery to remove the organs that make the hormones, such as the ovaries or testicles. Instead of radical surgery, the doctor can also use drugs to stop hormone production or change the way hormones work.

The side effects of hormone therapy can include nausea and vomiting. Hormone therapy can also bring about swelling or weight gain. In females, it may cause hot flashes, interrupted menstrual periods, and loss of fertility. In males, it may result in impotence or loss of fertility. These side effects can be temporary, long lasting, or permanent, depending on the situation. Questions to ask your doctor about hormone therapy are:

- Is surgery for removal of hormone-producing organs absolutely necessary, or can I alter hormone production with the help of drugs?
- What will the drugs do for and to me?
- Where will I be receiving the treatments?
- What are the side effects that I should expect, and which are permanent?
- Will I need to change what I eat and drink?

A similar methodology underlies a new cancer treatment called angiogenesis inhibitors therapy. Tumors require new blood vessels to supply them with oxygen and nutrients. This supply of nutrients allows them to grow and spread. Researchers have developed, and continue to experiment with, chemical compounds that inhibit—prevent or slow down—the growth of new blood vessels, thereby starving the tumor of what it needs to grow and spread.

Participating in Clinical Trials

Clinical trials are responsible for the advancement of cancer knowledge and treatment. They are basically cancer research studies in which promising new treatments are used on humans to make sure that the treatments are safe and effective.

The discovery of a new cancer treatment begins in the laboratory. Scientists develop and test new ideas. When one seems promising, it may be tested on animals. The results of a treatment tested in tissue samples can be very different from the results of that same treatment tested in living organisms. If the treatment works well with animals, the next stage is to administer it to a small group of humans with cancer.

If a human trial indicates that a new treatment may prove both safe and effective, the treatment becomes standard. Many of the treatments that are standard today are based on the successes of previous clinical trials. The downside of taking part in a clinical trial is that an experimental treatment may have unknown risks, and there is no guarantee that the treatment will produce good results. However, if a new treatment is proven effective, the patients that took part in the clinical trial are the first to benefit from it.

In clinical trials, there are strict guidelines for treatment and patient care that must be followed. They require that the doctor make a protocol. The protocol is a plan that explains everything that the study will be doing and why. The plan is then shown to the committee at the hospital or study site. The committee is made up of health professionals, clergy, and consumers. It will reject any protocol that will expose patients to extreme or careless risks.

Once a patient has decided to take part in a clinical trial, he or she must meet certain requirements in order to qualify. What makes a patient qualified is different for each trial. Some factors that can qualify a person may include age, gender, and cancer type and stage.

The number of patients involved in a clinical trial varies according to what phase it is in. There are three general phases of trials. A Phase I trial is the very first time a new treatment is tested on humans. It usually involves only a small number of patients because the risks of the new treatment in humans are still unknown. Doctors prefer to use patients who cannot be helped by other standard treatments. They look for the best way to administer the treatment and watch for any harmful side effects that it produces in humans. Phase II focuses on whether or not the drug has an effect on cancer in humans. Phase III trials include the largest number of patients. Treatments that get to Phase III have shown promise in the other two phases and have caused patients no obvious harm.

Doctors compare the results for patients who receive standard treatments with the results for those who receive the new treatment. Since the number of patients

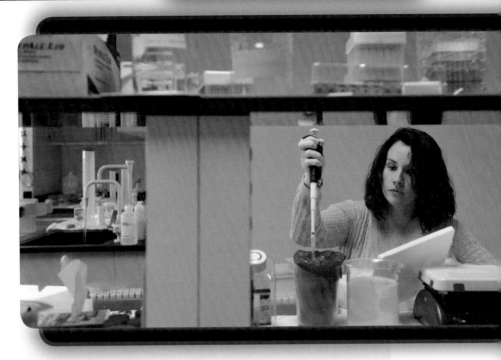

New tests, research, and studies on cancer and its treatment are being conducted everyday worldwide. This has led to new and more effective drugs, improved treatment therapies, and a better understanding of the disease and its progress, resulting in enhanced prevention, detection, and diagnosis.

needed for a Phase III trial is usually a set number, a computer is used to randomly decide who will receive the new treatment versus the standard treatment. This guarantees that everyone who wishes to take part in a clinical trial has equal chances of being chosen to receive the new treatment. Patients who receive the standard treatment are treated with the same effort and care as the ones who receive the new treatment.

There are some questions that you should ask your doctor if you are considering taking part in a clinical trial. Ask what the purpose of the trial is, who is sponsoring it, what you will be asked to do, what benefits can be expected from the treatment, what are the known potential risks and side effects of the treatment, and how it compares to the other standard treatment choices. You should also ask if you will have to pay for the treatment and how much of the costs will be picked up by your insurance company. If a patient participates in a clinical trial and has a bad reaction to the treatment, he or she is immediately given standard treatment instead. All patients who take part in a clinical trial have the right to leave at any time, for any reason.

MYTH

Being treated for cancer forces you to quit work or school and spend most of your time away from home in a hospital.

FACT

Most people with cancer are now treated on an outpatient basis in clinics and hospitals in their local community. In addition, treatment of the symptoms related to cancer treatment—such as nausea and diarrhea—has greatly improved, making normal life outside the house possible, including school and work.

MYTH

Getting a needle biopsy or surgically removing part or all of a tumor can actually cause cancer to spread to other parts of the body.

FACT

Surgical removal of a tumor cannot cause the cancer to spread. In fact, surgical removal is often the first and most important treatment of cancer. For most types of cancer, there is no evidence that a needle biopsy can disturb cancer cells and cause them to spread farther. Yet for some cancers, like testicular cancer, doctors avoid performing needle biopsies, instead opting to remove the suspected cancerous testicle.

MYTH

Each type of cancer requires a standard form of treatment for all patients.

FACT

A patient's cancer treatment is uniquely tailored to that person and is based on where the cancer is, if and how much it has spread, the patient's general state of health, and his or her genetic makeup.

MYTHS AND FACTS

CHAPTER 8

WHEN TREATMENT FAILS

Two of the more frightening aspects of being diagnosed with cancer are the fact that it can recur and that there are certain kinds of cancer that are considered terminal, meaning the cancer will be the cause of the patient's death.

WHEN CANCER RECURS

When cancer comes back, or recurs, patients may experience the same range of emotions that they felt when they were first diagnosed. Recurrent cancer is caused when a few cancer cells remain in the body after the first treatment. A recurrent cancer is not a new cancer. It is made of the same type of cancer cells as the original tumor. It can be found in parts of the body other than the original site, but it is still made of the same cancer cells and is called by the same name as the original or primary cancer.

Many of the tests used in the original diagnosis of the cancer are also used to diagnose the recurrent cancer. Similar treatments are also used in treating recurrent cancer. Patients with recurrent cancer should proceed much as they did when they first suspected they had cancer in terms of doctor's visits, promoting good physical and mental health, boosting the immune

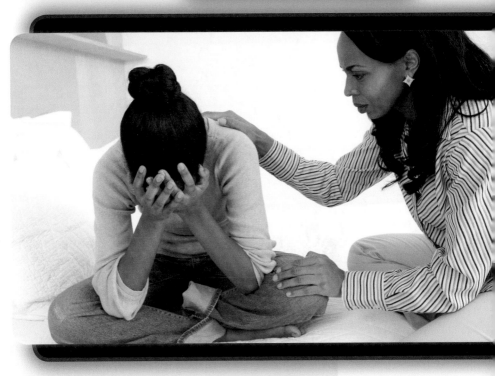

A cancer recurrence can be emotionally devastating. But it must be beaten back with the same energy, courage, care, and optimism that were brought to the first fight.

system, practicing relaxation techniques, seeking the support of friends and family, and maintaining a positive outlook and attitude.

WHEN TERMINAL CANCER IS DIAGNOSED

The diagnosis of terminal cancer means that, barring unforeseen circumstances, the disease will cause the end

ASK DR. JAN, PSYCHOLOGIST

First Name: Samantha

Question:

My mother just told my family and me that she has breast cancer. I feel terrified for both her and myself. How can I deal with my fear that she is going to die? How can I be there for my mom without letting her know that I'm so scared of her cancer and what may happen?

Answer:

A good place to start is to educate yourself about breast cancer. You may feel reassured by what you learn. Too often, when we hear the word "cancer," we think of it as a death sentence. The truth is that most patients diagnosed with breast cancer survive the illness. In addition, the percentage of those surviving breast cancer has generally increased over time, with improved diagnoses and treatment options.

Even so, it's still understandable to be scared, and it's true that not everyone does survive. While it may be difficult, it's important to share your feelings. If you think that's something you can do with your mom directly, that's great. Your mom may also want to have this conversation with you, and this would be a way to help her get it started. If you feel that it might be hard to do or too much for your mom, consider sharing your feelings with other family members, adults, or friends that you trust. This is a challenge for your mom but also for yourself and others who love her. You need to be supported as well.

We do know that a person's emotional state can have a very positive effect on his or her physical health. For this reason, it is important to try and help your mom feel optimistic about her chances for survival. Even in challenging situations where people do have terminal illnesses, learning ways to reduce stress and feel better emotionally can extend their lifetime and improve their quality of life. Challenges like these are often good reminders to not take each other for granted and to really try and enjoy our time together with friends and family. Take this opportunity to spend quality time with your mom now and in the future.

For more information on breast cancer and other cancers, visit the American Cancer Society's Web site, at http://www.cancer.org.

Ask a Question

Do you have a question that you would like answered? E-mail your question to Dr. Jan at drjan@rosenpub.com. If your question is selected, it will appear on the Teen Health & Wellness Web site in "Dr. Jan's Corner."

If you have an urgent question on a health or wellness issue, we strongly encourage you to call a hotline to speak to a qualified professional or speak to a trusted adult, such as a parent, teacher, or guidance counselor. You can find hotlines listed in the For More Information section of this book, or at www.teenhealthandwellness.com/static/hotlines.

of life for the patient. What should be emphasized, in cases of terminal cancer, is that a prognosis is a prediction. It is an estimate of the typical outcome of a patient's cancer, based on that person's age and general health and the cancer's type, location, and stage. Many people who were given a prognosis of terminal cancer live far longer than expected. Some even live to a normal life expectancy, though this is not typical.

A number of patients who outlive their prognosis have given themselves reasons for why they cannot allow the cancer to be terminal. This does not mean that you can think cancer away. Rather, it simply means that these people have a strong will to live, and this drive seems to assist the body's fight against the disease. These patients are actively enhancing whatever time they have left with life goals that extend beyond the limits of what terminal cancer typically allows. They are not letting cancer get in the way of their lives or the way they live them.

Terminal cancer is commonly referred to as advanced cancer and end-stage disease. People with advanced cancers face many challenges in their daily lives. One recurring challenge is thinking about the future. This is an overwhelming activity for anyone, not just patients with advanced cancer, because the future cannot be controlled, seen clearly, or planned for with a high degree of accuracy or certainty. What can be controlled is how we try to live each day. It may be helpful for terminal cancer patients to develop their own inspirational sayings or mottos. It is good to have a saying that can be repeated each day, for both comfort and motivation. An example is the following Sanskrit proverb about the importance of living each day as fully as possible:

Even if the news from your doctor is not encouraging, you must live each day to its fullest and celebrate your life from moment to moment.

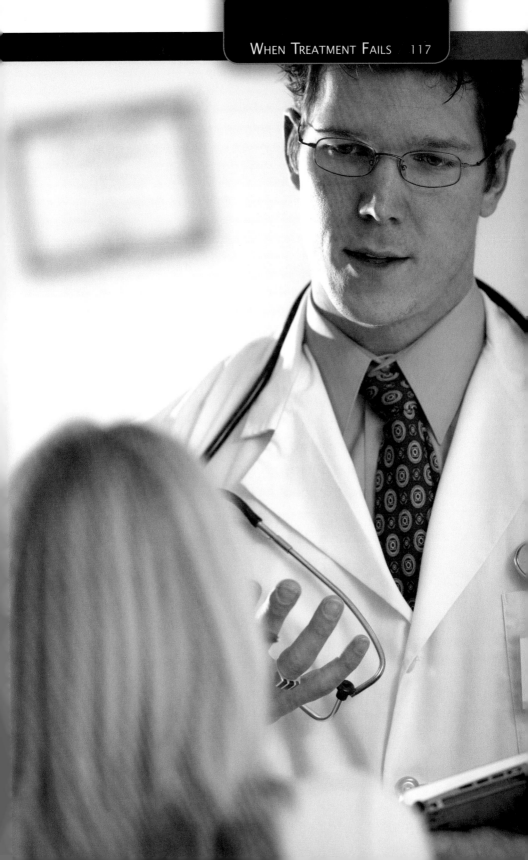

Yesterday is already a dream.
Tomorrow is only a vision.
But today—well lived—makes every yesterday a
dream of happiness, and every tomorrow a vision
of hope.

Many patients faced with terminal illnesses come to terms with their emotions by examining their beliefs about life and death. Others, bogged down with anxious thoughts and grief, can lose the will to live. Grief is a normal emotion when dealing with the idea of death, and patients should be encouraged to express their grief anytime they experience it. They need to work through their grief, rather than hang on to it. After grief can come the peace of acceptance, or a new understanding of how you want to live the rest of your life. The National Cancer Institute quotes a patient faced with the prospect of terminal cancer in its booklet on advanced cancers:

We can choose to wait for death, or we can choose
to live until we die.
Knowing that death is in the near future is no
   reason
to give up on the life we have today.

CHAPTER 9

LIFE AFTER CANCER TREATMENT

For patients who have undergone cancer treatment and are in remission or have been declared cured, life after cancer is really about living each day with a new understanding about themselves. Many patients have a new zest for life and take more chances than they did before developing cancer. Others try to enjoy and make the most of every moment, even if this is something as simple as sitting in the backyard and listening to birds sing or watching dogs play. However, patients in remission are still not free of concerns relating to cancer.

Going through cancer treatment can teach a person how to take excellent care of his or her health. Once treatment has brought about a remission, it is important that the patient keep working on maintaining good health. After all, why go through treatment to rid the body of cancer if you are just going to squander the good results that you have achieved? The long-term health needs of a patient in remission differ from person to person. Your doctor will give you an idea of your health needs and what you need to do in order to ensure good health in both the short-term and long-term. These guidelines should be followed closely to insure that you make the most of your return to health and help prevent a cancer recurrence or development of other diseases or illnesses.

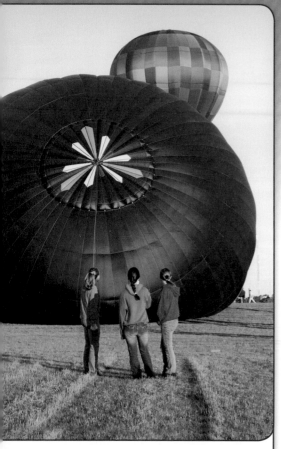

Surviving cancer can be a great inspiration to live your life more passionately, pursuing the dreams you once put on hold or shied away from.

Living Life, but Maintaining Vigilance

A cancer survivor is a person who has been diagnosed with, treated for, and is in remission from cancer. Cancer survivors who take an active role in maintaining their health need to get regular checkups, watch for warning signs, and adopt and maintain good health habits. After the conclusion of cancer treatments, patients should see their doctors about every three months. As time passes and the recovery progresses without any recurrences or other health problems, your doctor may indicate that annual or semiannual visits are fine.

There are certain symptoms that may be experienced if cancer recurs. The specific symptoms depend on the particular cancer the patient has had. Cancer survivors learn about these symptoms and watch for them. There are also long-term effects of certain treatments that can occur after treatment is finished. In addition, there are signs that survivors watch for that might mean other cancers have developed elsewhere in the body. With early detection, recurring or new cancers can often be controlled.

After cancer treatment, the body often experiences changes. These changes should not be interpreted as danger signs. Your doctor will explain how often to come in for checkups, what the warning signs are for cancer recurrence, the long-term side effects of cancer treatments, and the changes to expect in the body. Two important things to ask your doctor are what is the best diet to follow post-treatment and what is the best way to contact him or her if you have concerns.

MAINTAINING THE IMMUNE SYSTEM

Your immune system can take quite a beating during cancer treatment. It is important to keep it strong. With a strong immune system, the body can fight harder, more efficiently, and more effectively for good health. The immune system is weakened during treatment because infection-fighting white blood cells can be destroyed along with the cancer cells. With fewer white blood cells, the chances of developing infections increase.

When the white blood cell count is lower than normal, it is very important to try to prevent infections or

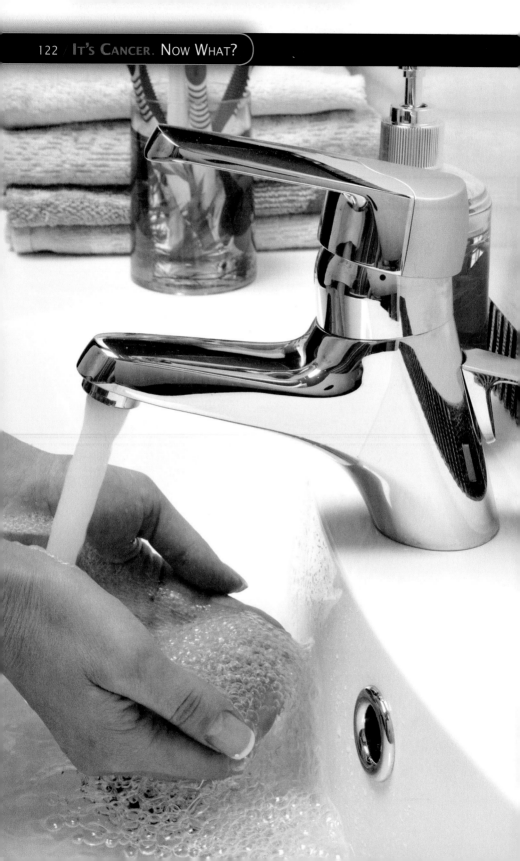

lessen their impact. The following is a list of steps that you should take to boost your immune system and reduce the risk of getting an infection during cancer treatment:

- Wash your hands often throughout the day. Always wash them before you eat and before and after using the bathroom.

- Avoid contact with people who are ill, and avoid going to crowded public places unnecessarily.

- Do not take any other medications (including aspirin) without first checking with your doctor.

- Do not drink any alcohol.

- Avoid activities that can lead to injuries.

- Take a warm bath, shower, or sponge bath every day. Lightly pat yourself dry.

- See your dentist before cancer treatment, rather than during or shortly after.

- Use a soft toothbrush and gentle toothpaste that won't hurt your gums. Brush your teeth and gums

Washing hands frequently will help reduce infections that are common to cancer patients whose immune systems are weakened by treatments.

after every meal, and rinse your toothbrush well after each use.

- Don't pick at your skin or the cuticles of your nails.

- Leave pimples and scratches alone.

- Use an electric shaver instead of a razor. This can prevent cuts in your skin.

- Be careful not to cut or nick yourself when handling scissors, needles, and sharp knives and tools.

- Clean any cuts or scrapes immediately with warm water, soap, and an antiseptic (a cleanser that kills germs).

- Use lotion to soften and heal your skin when it is dry and cracked.

- Use protective gloves when doing any yard work or cleaning up after pets.

- Clean your rectal area gently after each bowel movement.

- When blowing your nose, do it very gently into a soft tissue.

- Avoid children who have recently received immunization shots.

Your doctor needs to know right away if you experience any of the following symptoms just before, during, or soon after cancer treatments. They are signs of an infection and need to be addressed immediately:

- Fever (when the temperature is above 100°F [37.7°C])
- Sweating
- Chills
- Severe coughing or sore throat
- Diarrhea
- Burning sensation when you urinate
- Unusual vaginal discharge or itching
- Redness or tenderness, especially around any wounds, sores, or pimples

You should also let your doctor know any time that you experience side effects during cancer treatment. Ask your doctor for a list of expected and possible side effects related to your specific treatment. This will help you know what to expect and determine what side effects are considered to be normal and which are abnormal.

THE MOST IMPORTANT PERSON: YOU!

Even following successful treatment, survivors still experience a lot of anxiety when it comes to cancer. The important thing is for cancer survivors to deal with their emotions in whatever way works best for

SYMPTOMS OF INFECTION

Surviving cancer can recalibrate your priorities and help simplify your life, allowing you to shed annoyances, stresses, bad habits, and entanglements that held you back and compromised your health.

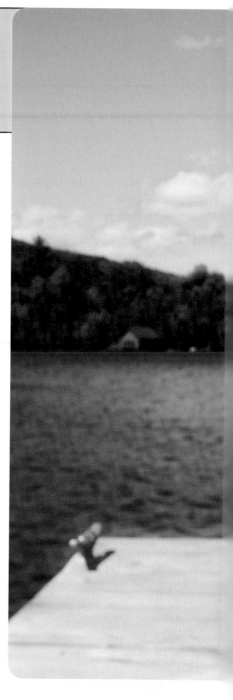

them. Something as seemingly harmless as a cold can make a survivor worry that cancer has come back or will come back. As the time nears for a checkup, survivors can experience stress. To ease this tension, they can use the same relaxation techniques that they practiced during treatment. They can also attend support groups whose members are cancer survivors.

Survivors must remember that even though they might be incredibly giving people, they need to take care of themselves first. They have to learn to say no to others when they don't want to do something, especially if they don't have the time, energy, or inclination.

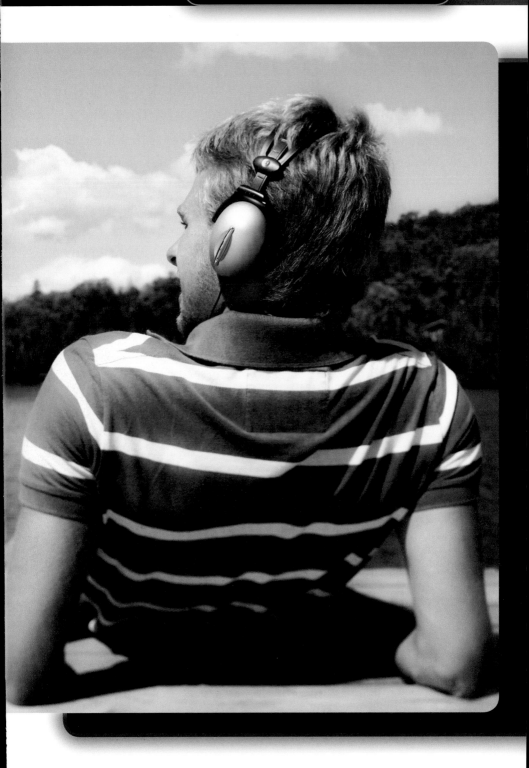

Having cancer has given you the right to respect yourself, your time, your health, and your happiness in ways that most people never learn to do in their entire lives. Try to think of this as a gift. Your experience with cancer and its cure should allow you to make healthier lifestyle choices and make your physical, mental, and emotional well-being the first priority. The new perspective you have gained can help minimize petty frustrations and stresses that wear on the body and mind. You now know what is truly important and essential in life. Focus on these things and live fully in the moment, creating dreams of happiness and visions of hope. Celebrate the life you have been given and your courage in living it to the hilt!

ABOUT DR. JAN

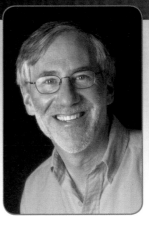

Dr. Jan Hittelman is a licensed psychologist with over twenty years of experience working with teens, children, adults, and families in a variety of settings.

In addition to clinical practices in California, Colorado, and New York, he has specialized in program development in partnership with school systems, psychiatric hospitals, correctional facilities and the courts, outpatient settings, residential treatment facilities, and private nonprofit organizations.

He founded Compass House, a nonprofit counseling collaborative for teens and their families. He launched Boulder Psychological Services in 2007.

Dr. Hittelman also authors a monthly newspaper column entitled "Surviving the Teenage Years" in the *Boulder Daily Camera*, writes monthly columns for the Boulder Valley School District under the sponsorship of the Parent Engagement Network, and publishes an online question-and-answer column for teens in the Rosen Publishing Group's online resource Teen Health & Wellness.

Teen Health & Wellness: Real Life, Real Answers (*http://www.teenhealthandwellness.com*) is a database designed for teens on issues relating to health, fitness, alcohol, drugs, mental health, family life, and much more. Check your school or local library for access.

GLOSSARY

adjunctive therapy Anticancer drugs or hormones given after surgery and/or radiation to help prevent the cancer from coming back.

administer To give out in doses.

alopecia Hair loss.

anemia Having a low number of red blood cells. Symptoms of anemia include feeling tired, weak, and short of breath.

anesthetic A numbing substance that causes a temporary loss of sensation or feeling, including pain.

benign Noncancerous.

biological therapy Treatment to stimulate or restore the ability of the immune system to fight infection; also called immunotherapy.

biopsy The removal and examination of tissue for the purpose of diagnosis.

bone marrow The spongy inner tissue of bones where blood cells are made.

bone marrow transplant Procedure in which a patient receives marrow from a donor in order to restore blood cells after receiving radiation and/or chemotherapy treatments strong enough to kill all cancer cells.

cancer General term for more than one hundred diseases in which abnormal cells grow out of control, damage healthy cells, and spread to other parts of the body.

carcinogen A chemical or other substance that can cause cancer.

carcinoma Cancer of the tissues that line or cover the body surface or organs.

chemoprevention The use of chemicals and drugs to lower a person's chances of developing certain kinds of cancer.

chemotherapy The use of drugs and chemicals to treat cancer.

clinical trial An experimental study conducted on volunteers. Each study is designed to answer scientific questions and find new, better ways of preventing or treating cancer.

combination chemotherapy The use of more than one drug to treat cancer.

curative Treatment aimed at bringing about a cure for cancer.

diagnosis The identification of the presence of a disease.

gene The basic unit of inheritance in a body's cells.

grade A determination of how closely cancer cells resemble normal tissue; it is used to predict the rate at which cancer cells are likely to grow.

hematologist A doctor who specializes in blood diseases.

hormone The natural substance released by an organ that influences the function of other organs in the body.

injection The use of a syringe, or needle, to push fluids or drugs into the body; often called a shot.

intravenous (IV) The method of introducing medications into the body through a vein.

malignant Cancerous.

metastasis The spread of cancer from its first, or primary, tumor to other parts of the body.

oncogene A gene that, when mutated or present at high levels, can help turn a normal cell into a cancer cell.

oncologist A doctor who specializes in treating cancer.

oncology The science of preventing, treating, and diagnosing cancer.

palliative Treatment to relieve the symptoms of cancer.

pathologist A doctor who specializes in the study of cells and tissues that have been removed from the body by biopsy or surgery.

platelet The blood cell that helps stop bleeding by clotting at the wound.

predisposition The state of being favorable or open to something beforehand; to have a tendency toward something.

prognosis An estimate or prediction of the outcome of a disease, such as cancer.

protocol A general treatment plan.

radiation A process in which energetic particles or waves travel through a medium or space. As a cancer treatment, radiation is used to control malignant cells.

radiation therapy Cancer treatment with high-energy rays.

radiologist A doctor specializing in the making of diagnostic medical images of areas inside the body. The images are made with X-rays, sound waves, and other types of energy.

recurrence The redevelopment of cancer in the body after an earlier cancer has been treated.

red blood cell The blood cell that supplies oxygen to tissues of the body.

remission The partial or complete disappearance of signs and symptoms of cancer.

risk factor Something that increases a person's chance of developing a disease.

sarcoma A cancer of the connective tissue of the body, such as bone and cartilage.

side effect A physical problem that results from treatment.

stage A classification of a patient's cancer that takes into account the location of the primary tumor, the size and number of tumors, the spread of cancer into lymph nodes, the cell type, the tumor grade, and the presence or absence of metastasis.

suppress To prevent the development or expression of.

surgery A procedure in which the body is opened medically; also called an operation.

symptom A reaction that is a sign of an illness.

treatment Medical therapy to bring about a remission or cure.

tumor A mass of tissue composed of an abnormal growth of cells. Tumors can be benign or malignant.

tumor suppressor gene A gene that slows or stops the growth of tumors.

white blood cell The blood cell that fights infection.

FOR MORE INFORMATION

American Cancer Society (ACS)
250 Williams Street NW
Atlanta, GA 30303
(800) 227-2345
Web site: http://www.cancer.org

The ACS is a nationwide, community-based health organization dedicated to eliminating cancer as a major health problem. It has thirteen chartered divisions and more than 3,400 local offices.

American Public Health Association (APHA)
800 I Street NW
Washington, DC 20001
(202) 777-2742
Web site: http://www.apha.org

The APHA is an organization of health professionals dedicated to improving public health.

CancerCare National Office
275 Seventh Avenue, Floor 22
New York, NY 10001
(800) 813-HOPE (4673)
Web site: http://www.cancercare.org

CancerCare has over a hundred staff members who help more than 100,000 people each year face the crisis of cancer. CancerCare's National Office serves people with cancer and their loved ones throughout the entire fifty states, Puerto Rico, and the U.S. Virgin Islands. By using the phone and Internet, CancerCare social workers can help people no matter where they are.

Centers for Disease Control and Prevention (CDC)

1600 Clifton Road
Atlanta, GA 30333
(800) 232-4636
Web site: http://www.cdc.gov

The CDC is an organization that provides the public with reliable information about diseases and other health-related topics.

Health Canada

Address Locator 0900C2
Ottawa, ON K1A 0K9
Canada
(866) 225-0709
Web site: http://www.hc-sc.gc.ca

Health Canada is the federal department that is responsible for help-ing Canadians maintain and improve their health. Its goal is for Canada to be among the countries with the healthiest people in the world.

International Union Against Cancer (UICC)

World Cancer Campaign
62 Route de Frontenex
1207 Geneva, Switzerland
Web site: http://www.worldcancercampaign.org

The International Union Against Cancer (UICC) initiated the World Cancer Campaign in 2005. Since 2006, UICC has coordinated World Cancer Day activities (Feb. 4), supported by members, part-ners, the World Health Organization, the International Atomic Energy Agency, and other international bodies. This program aims to raise awareness about the ways we can prevent cancer through the choices we make, including creating smoke-free environments, being "sun smart," engaging in healthy diets and physical activity, and preventing cancer-related infections.

Johns Hopkins Hospital

600 North Wolfe Street

Baltimore, MD 21287

(410) 955-5000

Web site: http://www.hopkinsmedicine.org

The mission of Johns Hopkins is to improve the health of the community and the world by setting the standard of excellence in medical education, research, and clinical care.

Mayo Clinic

200 First Street SW

Rochester, MN 55905

(507) 284-2511

Web site: http://www.mayoclinic.org

The Mayo Clinic is a leader in translating knowledge gained from cancer research into effective care for cancer patients and their families. It is the first and largest integrated, not-for-profit group practice in the world.

Memorial Sloan-Kettering Cancer Center

1275 York Avenue

New York, NY 10065

(212) 639-2000

Web site: http://www.mskcc.org

The world's oldest and largest private cancer center, Memorial Sloan-Kettering has devoted more than a century to patient care as well as to innovative research, making significant contributions to new and better therapies for the treatment of cancer.

National Cancer Institute (NCI)

Office of Communications and Education
Public Inquiries Office
6116 Executive Boulevard, Suite 300
Bethesda, MD 20892-8322
Web site: http://www.cancer.gov

The NCI is part of the National Institutes of Health (NIH), one of eleven agencies that comprise the Department of Health and Human Services (HHS). It is the federal government's principal agency for cancer research and training.

Public Health Agency of Canada

1015 Arlington Street
Winnipeg, MB R3E 3R2
Canada
(204) 789-2000
Web site: http://www.phac-aspc.gc.ca

The Public Health Agency of Canada is a government organization that promotes health and helps people prevent and control diseases, injuries, and infections.

WEB SITES

Due to the changing nature of Internet links, Rosen Publishing has developed an online list of Web sites related to the subject of this book. This site is updated regularly. Please use this link to access the list:

http://www.rosenlinks.com/411/can

FOR FURTHER READING

Altschuler, Lise N., and Karolyn A. Gazella. *The Definitive Guide to Cancer: An Integrative Approach to Prevention, Treatment, and Healing.* 3rd ed. Berkeley, CA: Celestial Arts, 2010.

Anderson, Greg. *Cancer: 50 Essential Things to Do.* 3rd ed. New York, NY: Plume, 2009.

Barnard, Neal D., and Jennifer K. Riley. *The Cancer Survivor's Guide: Foods That Help You Fight Back.* Summertown, TN: Healthy Living Publications, 2009.

Becton, Randy. *Everyday Strength: A Cancer Patient's Guide to Spiritual Survival.* Grand Rapids, MI: Baker Books, 2006.

Beliveau, Richard, and Denis Gingras. *Foods to Fight Cancer: Essential Foods to Help Prevent Cancer.* New York, NY: DK Adult, 2007.

Canfield, Jack, Mark Victor Hansen, and David Tabatsky. *Chicken Soup for the Soul: The Cancer Book: 101 Stories of Courage, Support, and Love.* Cos Cob, CT: Chicken Soup for the Soul Publishing, 2009.

Katz, Rebecca, and Mat Edelson. *The Cancer-Fighting Kitchen: Nourishing, Big Flavor Recipes for Cancer Treatment and Recovery.* Berkeley, CA: Celestial Arts, 2009.

Keane, Maureen. *What to Eat If You Have Cancer: Healing Foods That Boost Your Immune System.* New York, NY: McGraw-Hill, 2006.

McKay, Judith, and Tamera Schacher. *The Chemotherapy Survival Guide: Everything You Need to Know to Get Through Treatment.* Oakland, CA: New Harbinger Publications, 2009.

Ortega, Yvonne. *Hope for the Journey Through Cancer: Inspiration for Each Day.* Grand Rapids, MI: Revell, 2007.

Servan-Schreiber, David. *Anti-Cancer: A New Way of Life.* New York, NY: Viking, 2009.

Silver, Julie K. *What Helped Get Me Through: Cancer Survivors Share Wisdom and Hope.* Atlanta, GA: American Cancer Society, 2008.

INDEX

A

abnormal cells, 9, 23, 25, 30, 93
abscesses, 10–11
adenocarcinoma, 12–13
adjunctive therapy, 90, 104–105
alcohol, 14, 19, 24, 27, 31, 34, 37, 44–45, 123
anesthesia, 56, 58, 92
anger, 63, 66, 67–68, 72
anxiety, 26, 55, 63, 72, 73, 75, 91, 125–128

B

bacteria, 15, 16, 19, 21
biological therapy, 90, 100–102
biopsies, 54, 56, 88, 111
bladder, 35, 47
blood tests, 54, 55–56, 61
blood vessels, 11, 12, 13, 107
bone marrow, 12 , 58–59
  samples, 58–59
  transplants, 90, 102–104
bones, 12, 13, 15, 93, 100
bone scans, 59–60
brain, 60, 101

breast cancer, 15, 26–27, 37, 45, 48, 52, 59, 62, 101, 105, 114, 115
breast exam, 52–53

C

cancer
  causes, 6, 23–31
  coping with, 6, 63–82
  facts, 14, 111
  mechanics of, 7–9
  naming, 12, 15
  prevention, 5, 6, 34–53
  recovery, 75, 119–128
  recurrence, 112–113, 121
  risk factors, 6, 31–33, 37
  staging and grading, 14, 83, 86–88
  symptoms, 23, 51–52
  terminal, 112, 113, 115–118
  tests and screening for, 36–37, 54–62
  treating, 4–5, 6, 19, 22, 24, 69, 71, 75, 82–85, 88, 89–110, 119, 121
carcinogens, 23–24, 25, 27, 28, 29, 32, 35, 37, 39, 43
carcinomas, 12–13
cartilage, 12, 13
cell reproduction, 7–8, 30

cervical cancer, 33, 35, 37, 47, 48, 59, 62, 93, 101
charred foods, 24, 43
checkups, 27, 31, 32, 36–37, 46, 50, 120, 121
chemoprevention, 62
chemotherapy, 90, 96–100, 102, 103, 104, 105
cholesterol-lowering drugs, 24
clinical trials, 107–109
colon, 11, 12, 35, 36, 37, 43, 45, 48, 58, 61, 62, 101
computed tomography (CT) scan, 57
counseling, 65, 73–75, 84
cryosurgery, 93

D

denial, 63, 65
depression, 19, 63, 66, 70
dermatologists, 45
DNA, 29, 61, 93, 101
Dr. Jan, questions for, 26–27, 40–41, 66–67, 114–115

E

electroencephalogram (EEG), 60
endoscopies, 57–58, 61
epithelial tissue, 12
esophagus, 35, 45, 47, 60
exercise, 20, 27, 31, 35, 48, 69, 92

F

fat, body, 12, 13
fat, in food, 31, 39, 42, 44
fear, 63, 66, 68, 72, 91–92

G

genes, 8, 18, 27–30, 48, 61, 101–102
genetic counselors, 30
genetics, and disease, 14, 19, 25–28, 30, 31, 32, 61
guilt, 70–71

H

heart disease, 34, 35, 39
hematologist, 88
hepatitis B, 35, 44
HIV, 15, 18, 35
hope, 65, 72, 75
hormone therapy, 90, 105–107
human papillomavirus (HPV), 33, 35

I

immune system, 12, 15, 16–18
  maintaining, 121–124
  things that strengthen, 19–22
  things that weaken, 18–19, 69, 71, 99
immunologists, 21

infection, symptoms of, 125
inherited risk factors, 32
in situ cancer, 87
invasive cancer, 87

K

kidneys, 47, 101

L

larynx, 35, 45, 47
laser therapy, 93
leukemias, 12, 59, 101
liposarcoma, 13
liver, 13, 15, 44, 45, 62,
    93, 101
loneliness, 19, 71–72
lungs, 12, 15, 25, 34, 35, 47,
    62, 93, 99, 101
lymphatic system, 12, 15, 60
lymphatic vessels, 11
lymph nodes, 15, 52, 60, 86,
    87, 91
lymphocytes (white blood
    cells), 15, 18, 80, 96, 99,
    102, 121
lymphomas, 12, 101

M

magnetic resonance imaging
    (MRI), 57
mammographies, 27, 59, 61
markers, 55–56
medical team, 82–85,
    88–89, 111
meditation, 20, 69

metastasis, 11, 86, 87
molecules, 16–18
moles, 9, 46, 47
mononucleosis, 15
mouth, 35, 37, 45, 47, 62
muscle, 11, 12, 15

N

nonself signal, 18, 21, 22
nutrition, as disease preven-
    tion, 14, 20, 39, 42–44, 48

O

obesity, 27, 35, 48
oncogenes, 28–30
oncologists, 5, 88
ovarian cancer, 48, 62, 101

P

pancreas, 35, 47, 101
Pap tests, 59, 61
pathologist, 88
polyps, 11, 60
precancerous growths, 11, 36
prostate gland, 12, 37, 43,
    48, 56, 62, 93, 101, 105
proteins, 22, 29, 30

R

radiation, 24, 28, 29, 31, 32,
    48–49
    therapy, 88, 90, 91, 93–96,
    102, 103, 104, 105
radiation oncologist, 88

radiologist, 88–89
radon, 49
rectal cancer, 37, 43, 45, 61, 62, 101
red blood cells, 13, 55, 56
relaxation techniques, 20, 80–82, 113, 126
remission, 89, 119
research, 83

S

sarcomas, 12
second opinions, 83–84
self-examinations, 46–47, 52–53
sleep, 19, 20
skin cancer, 35–36, 37, 46, 62, 93
smoking, 14, 20, 24, 25, 31, 32–33, 34–35, 37–39, 40–41, 45, 47
stomach, 12, 15, 43, 60, 61, 62
stress, 19, 26, 69–70, 80
sun, 14, 31, 36, 37, 46–47
sun protection factor (SPF), 46
support
  building a network of, 70–71, 75–77, 80, 126

providing to someone with cancer, 63–64, 66–67, 76, 78–79
surgery, 10, 50, 56, 62, 88, 90–93, 104, 106, 111

T

talking, to deal with cancer, 6, 65, 68, 71–73, 76–77
testicular cancer, 62
tumors, 23, 28, 30, 60, 106, 111, 112
  benign, 9–11, 52, 57
  malignant, 11–12, 56, 57, 86, 88, 90–91, 92, 94, 95
tumor suppressor genes, 28, 30

U

urine tests, 54, 56

V

viruses, 16, 19, 21

X

X-rays, 24, 48–49, 54, 56–57, 59, 60, 89, 95

About the Authors

Luke Graham is a writer who lives in Lambertville, New Jersey.

Henrietta M. Lily is a writer who lives and works in New York. She is daily and personally inspired by some happy, healthy, and wonderful cancer survivors.

Photo Credits

Cover, p. 1 © www.istockphoto.com/Joseph Abbott; p. 4 blue jean images/Getty Images; p. 8 MedicalRF. com/Getty Images; pp. 10, 29, 87 NCI; p. 13 © Dr P. Marazzi/SCIENCE PHOTO LIBRARY/CMSP; p. 17 CMSP/Getty Images; p. 21 Kallista Images/Getty Images; pp. 24, 32, 36, 38, 45, 55, 64, 69, 113, 117, 120, 122, 126–127 Thinkstock.com; pp. 26, 40, 66, 114, 129 Courtesy of Jan S. Hittelman, Ph.D.; p. 49 © www.istockphotos.com/BanksPhotos; p. 58 Joos Mind/ Stone/Getty Images; p. 60 © 2005 Terese Winslow, U.S. Govt. has certain rights; p. 74 © Bryan Patrick/ Sacramento Bee/Zuma Press; p. 91 © B. Slaven/CMSP; p. 94 © M. Bradford/CMSP; p. 98 © Véronique Burger/ Photo Researchers, Inc.; p. 103 Joe Burbank/Orlando Sentinal/Newscom.com; p. 109 Jahi Chikwendiu/The Washington Post via Getty Images.

Photo Researcher: Amy Feinberg